Neck Rejuvenation

Editors

MARK M. HAMILTON
MARK M. BEATY

FACIAL PLASTIC SURGERY CLINICS OF NORTH AMERICA

www.facialplastic.theclinics.com

Consulting Editor
J. REGAN THOMAS

May 2014 • Volume 22 • Number 2

ELSEVIER

1600 John F. Kennedy Boulevard • Suite 1800 • Philadelphia, Pennsylvania 19103-2899

http://www.theclinics.com

FACIAL PLASTIC SURGERY CLINICS OF NORTH AMERICA Volume 22, Number 2
May 2014 ISSN 1064-7406, ISBN-13: 978-0-323-29705-9

Editor: Joanne Husovski
Developmental Editor: Susan Showalter

Facial Plastic Surgery Clinics of North America (ISSN 1064-7406) is published quarterly by Elsevier Inc., 360 Park Avenue South, New York, NY 10010-1710. Months of issue are February, May, August, and November. Business and Editorial Offices: 1600 John F. Kennedy Blvd., Suite 1800, Philadelphia, PA 19103-2899. Periodicals postage paid at New York, NY, and additional mailing offices. Subscription prices are $390.00 per year (US individuals), $525.00 per year (US institutions), $445.00 per year (Canadian individuals), $653.00 per year (Canadian institutions), $535.00 per year (foreign individuals), $653.00 per year (foreign institutions), $185.00 per year (US students), and $255.00 per year (foreign students). Foreign air speed delivery is included in all *Clinics* subscription prices. All prices are subject to change without notice. POSTMASTER: Send address changes to *Facial Plastic Surgery Clinics*, Elsevier Health Sciences Division, Subscription Customer Service, 3251 Riverport Lane, Maryland Heights, MO 63043. **Customer service: 1-800-654-2452 (US and Canada); 1-314-447-8871 (outside US and Canada); Fax: 314-447-8029; E-mail:journalscustomerservice-usa@elsevier.com (for print support); journalsonline support-usa@elsevier.com (for online support).**

Reprints. For copies of 100 or more of articles in this publication, please contact the Commercial Reprints Department, Elsevier Inc., 360 Park Avenue South, New York, NY 10010-1710. Tel.: 212-633-3874; Fax: 212-633-3820; E-mail: reprints@elsevier.com.

Facial Plastic Surgery Clinics of North America is covered in *MEDLINE/PubMed* (*Index Medicus*).

Contributors

CONSULTING EDITOR

J. REGAN THOMAS, MD, FACS
Professor and Chairman, Mansueto Professor
and Head of Department of Otolaryngology—
Head and Neck Surgery, University of Illinois at
Chicago, Chicago, Illinois

EDITORS

MARK M. HAMILTON, MD, FACS
Clinical Assistant Professor, Department of
Otolaryngology—Head and Neck Surgery,
Indiana University School of Medicine;
Hamilton Facial Plastic Surgery, Indianapolis,
Indiana

MARK M. BEATY, MD
President and Medical Director, Beaty Facial
Plastic Surgery, Alpharetta, Georgia

AUTHORS

STEWART I. ADAM, MD
Chief Resident, Section of Otolaryngology,
Head and Neck Surgery, Department of
Surgery, Yale University School of Medicine,
New Haven, Connecticut

RAMI K. BATNIJI, MD, FACS
Batniji Facial Plastic Surgery, Newport Beach,
California

MARK M. BEATY, MD
President and Medical Director, Beaty Facial
Plastic Surgery, Alpharetta, Georgia

ROBERT W. BROBST, MD
Brobst Facial Plastic Surgery, Plano, Texas

DAVID CHAN, MD
Resident, Department of Otolaryngology—
Head and Neck Surgery, Indiana University
School of Medicine, Indianapolis, Indiana

TATIANA K. DIXON, MD
Assistant Professor, Facial Plastic &
Reconstructive Surgery/General

Otolaryngology, Department of
Otolaryngology—Head and Neck Surgery,
University of Illinois at Chicago, Chicago,
Illinois

J. KEVIN DUPLECHAIN, MD
Lafayette, Louisiana

LINDSAY EISLER, MD
Associate Professor, Department of
Otolaryngology—Head and Neck Surgery,
Geisinger Medical Center, Danville,
Pennsylvania

EDWARD FARRIOR, MD, FACS
Assistant Professor, Department of
Otolaryngology—Head and Neck
Surgery, University of South Florida,
Tampa, Florida

MARIA FERGUSON, BS, ME
Meridian Plastic Surgeons, Meridian Plastic
Surgery Center, Indianapolis, Indiana

NEIL A. GORDON, MD, FACS
Clinical Assistant Professor of Surgery, Director, Head and Neck, Aesthetic Surgery & Coordinator, Residency Education in Facial Plastic and Reconstructive Surgery, Section of Otolaryngology, Head and Neck Surgery, Department of Surgery, Yale University School of Medicine, New Haven; New England Surgical Center, The Retreat at Split Rock, Wilton, Connecticut

MARK M. HAMILTON, MD, FACS
Clinical Assistant Professor, Department of Otolaryngology—Head and Neck Surgery, Indiana University School of Medicine, Indianapolis; Hamilton Facial Plastic Surgery, Greenwood, Indiana

J. DAVID HOLCOMB, MD
Holcomb–Kreithen Plastic Surgery and MedSpa, Sarasota, Florida

ANDREW A. JACONO, MD
Facial Plastic and Reconstructive Surgery, North Shore University Hospital, Manhasset; Facial Plastic Surgery, The New York Eye and Ear Infirmary, New York; Department of Otorhinolaryngology, Head and Neck Surgery, The Albert Einstein College of Medicine, Bronx; Facial Plastic Surgery, The New York Center for Facial Plastic and Laser Surgery, New York, New York

STEPHEN W. PERKINS, MD, FACS
Clinical Associate Professor, Department of Otolaryngology—Head and Neck Surgery, Indiana University School of Medicine; President, Meridian Plastic Surgery Center, Indianapolis, Indiana

SCOTT SHADFAR, MD
Meridian Plastic Surgeons, Indianapolis, Indiana

BENJAMIN TALEI, MD
Facial Plastic Surgery, The New York Center for Facial Plastic and Laser Surgery New York, New York; Facial Plastic Surgery, The Beverly Hills Center for Plastic and Laser Surgery, Beverly Hills, California

J. REGAN THOMAS, MD, FACS
Professor and Chairman, Mansueto Professor and Head of Department of Otolaryngology—Head and Neck Surgery, University of Illinois at Chicago, Chicago, Illinois

HEATHER H. WATERS, MD
Meridian Plastic Surgery Center, Indianapolis, Indiana

HARRY V. WRIGHT, MD, MS
Associate Professor, Department of Otolaryngology—Head and Neck Surgery, University of South Florida, Tampa, Florida

Contents

Anatomy and Physiology of the Aging Neck   161

Scott Shadfar and Stephen W. Perkins

> This article discusses the surgically relevant anatomic and physiologic tenets of the aging neck. Procedures performed to rejuvenate and contour the aging neck can be challenging. A thorough understanding of the underlying neck anatomy, as well as the physiology associated with aging, is critical for surgical planning, execution, and achieving aesthetically pleasing outcomes. These topics are reviewed and used as the foundation for a discussion of various other techniques.

Preoperative Evaluation of the Aging Neck Patient   171

J. Regan Thomas and Tatiana K. Dixon

> The appearance of the neck plays an important role in terms of the patient's overall facial appearance. Facial rejuvenation procedures incorporate rejuvenation and improvement of the neck's appearance as a key component. Preoperative evaluation of the aging neck determines the type of rejuvenation procedures that will be required. There are key components of the neck that should be evaluated, assessed, and documented. Subsequently, appropriate treatment modalities may be incorporated into the operative or treatment plan. Key components include evaluation of the mandibular margin, hyoid position, condition of the skin, soft tissue adipose, and the status of the platysmal muscle layer.

A Progressive Approach to Neck Rejuvenation   177

Mark M. Beaty

> The progressive approach to neck and facial rejuvenation is a comprehensive method for evaluation and correction of common aging changes seen in the lower face and neck. The surgical results are natural in appearance, as the rejuvenation method chosen is specifically and continuously adjusted for optimal results throughout the evaluation and surgical process. The increased burden on the surgeon to master a variety of techniques and to develop the judgment needed to decide in a progressive manner which is the most appropriate for use in each patient is more than compensated for by improved results and greater patient satisfaction.

Noninvasive Treatment of the Neck   191

Robert W. Brobst, Maria Ferguson, and Stephen W. Perkins

 A video of Ulthera treatment accompanies this article

> Emerging trends in neck rejuvenation include the incorporation of nonsurgical treatment modalities as an offering to those patients desiring minimal downtime and accepting of mild results. Intense focused ultrasound is a promising technology for treatment of the neck. It is rapidly growing in clinical use and undergoing further investigation to determine optimum treatment parameters and make its outcomes more predictable.

digital imaging, and discussion of perioperative instructions are of utmost importance. Although many techniques exist, the modified deep plane extended superficial muscular aponeurotic system rhytidectomy with submentoplasty reliably delivers a significant improvement with lasting results.

The Deep-Plane Approach to Neck Rejuvenation

Neil A. Gordon and Stewart I. Adam

 A video of a complete extended deep-plane midface lift with platysma tightening accompanies the article

This article provides the facial plastic surgeon with anatomic and embryologic evidence to support the use of the deep-plane rhytidectomy for optimal treatment of the aging neck. An anatomic basis is established that demonstrates this technique's ability to maximize neck rejuvenation through its direct relationship to midface soft-tissue mobilization. A detailed description of the procedure, aimed at providing safe and consistent results, is presented with insights into anatomic landmarks, technical nuances, and alternative approaches to facial variations.

Vertical Neck Lifting

Andrew A. Jacono and Benjamin Talei

The authors' vertical neck lifting procedure is an extended deep plane facelift, which elevates the skin and SMAS-platysma complex as a composite unit. The goal is to redrape cervicomental laxity vertically onto the face rather than laterally and post-auricularly. The authors consider this an extended technique because it lengthens the deep plane flap from the angle of the mandible into the neck to release the cervical retaining ligaments that limit platysmal redraping. This technique does not routinely use midline platysmal surgery because it counteracts the extent of vertical redraping. A majority of aging face patients are good candidates for this procedure in isolation, but indications for combining vertical neck lifting with submental surgery are elucidated.

Complications/Sequelae of Neck Rejuvenation

Rami K. Batniji

Neck lift surgery performed in isolation or in conjunction with a facelift provides a more youthful cervicomental angle. Complications related to neck lift surgery vary from contour irregularities that may improve with time or conservative measures,to contour irregularities that persist and may benefit from delayed surgical intervention, to expanding hematomas that require immediate surgical intervention. This article reviews complications of neck lift surgery and their etiologies, methods to minimize the incidence of these complications, and management.

Index

FACIAL PLASTIC SURGERY CLINICS OF NORTH AMERICA

Preface
Neck Rejuvenation

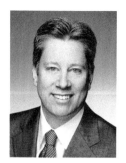
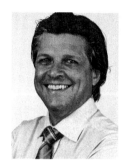

Mark M. Hamilton, MD, FACS   Mark M. Beaty, MD
Editors

It is an honor for us to serve as guest editors and to welcome you to this issue of *Facial Plastic Surgery Clinics of North America*. It has been a little over a century since the first procedures were performed and described for rejuvenation of the neck. Since that time, the pace of development and range of options available for aesthetic improvement of the neck have exponentially increased. Key concepts of facial structure including the nature of the SMAS and retaining ligaments of the face, enhanced methods of mobilization and fixation of supporting structures, and the importance of volume removal and enhancement for facial and neck contour have been described over decades by many innovative authors. This issue is devoted to bringing surgeons up-to-date on the latest concepts and techniques available to reverse the signs of aging in the neck.

Our issue begins by highlighting the important anatomy and background information to consider when approaching rejuvenation of the aging neck. We then explore a variety of approaches for cervicofacial rejuvenation by some of the thought leaders of our time. They present differing opinions on approaches and techniques, but all can claim and demonstrate outstanding results. Other important concepts addressed include fibrin sealants and other adjunctive procedures beyond lifting and resurfacing, a deeper look at the growing options in nonsurgical neck rejuvenation, and the role of laser fibers in contour correction and lifting. The authors have brought diverse and interesting ideas forward with critical assessments of their value and an honest look at potential downsides and complications.

Our patients continue to request neck rejuvenation as one of their top priorities. We hope this issue of *Facial Plastic Surgery Clinics of North America* will stimulate a personal assessment of new thoughts and approaches and help you give your patients the best results possible.

Mark M. Hamilton, MD, FACS
Hamilton Facial Plastic Surgery
Indianapolis, IN, USA

Mark M. Beaty, MD
Beaty Facial Plastic Surgery
Alpharetta, GA, USA

E-mail addresses:
mmckhamilton@gmail.com (M.M. Hamilton)
mmbeaty@comcast.net (M.M. Beaty)

Facial Plast Surg Clin N Am 22 (2014) ix
http://dx.doi.org/10.1016/j.fsc.2014.02.001
1064-7406/14/$ – see front matter

facialplastic.theclinics.com

Anatomy and Physiology of the Aging Neck

Scott Shadfar, MD[a], Stephen W. Perkins, MD[a,b],*

KEYWORDS

- Neck anatomy • Aging neck • Cervicomental angle • Platysma • Neck aesthetics • Cervicoplasty

KEY POINTS

- The skin's ability to conform to the newly contoured neck shape depends on the skin's inherent pliability and texture, and is often related to its elastin and collagen content, which diminishes with age.
- Thick-skinned and overweight patients should not expect dramatic, long-lasting results of their neck contouring procedure because of gravitational forces and the weight of the tissues.
- The platysma courses inferolateral to superomedial, with 3 variations in patterns of interdigitation or decussation in the midline submental region.
- Patients with minimal or no platysmal decussation can have interplatysmal fat in the submental region herniate between the medial edges, which is contiguous with the deep subplatysmal fat, further contributing to the appearance of neck aging.
- Bone resorption at the level of the mentum, mandibular body, and mandibular angle contribute to the clinical appearance of aging, with changes seen at the cervicomental angle as well as the overall superficial topography of the neck.

INTRODUCTION

Neck rejuvenation and contouring procedures continue to expand and evolve, with a multitude of techniques designed to address the clinical consequences related to aging. Patients present with concerns regarding the aged appearance of their neck, often caused by changes in skin quality, fat accumulation, muscle tone, sun damage, or changes after weight gain or loss.[1] The principal contouring techniques in neck rejuvenation are designed to transform specific regions of the neck by reduction and/or relocation of volume, redundancy, or laxity.[2] This article focuses on the respective anatomic levels of the neck, which allows a more systematic approach when evaluating and treating patients with signs of neck aging.

Anatomy and Physiology by Anatomic Structure

Patterns of aging are variable. Those patients with thin necks, good skeletal support, and good neck height age differently from those patients with heavy, short necks and poor mandibular support.[3] The superficial topography of the neck also affects the perception of a youthful or aged neck. The interplay of the structures deep to the skin, and the skin's ability to drape over them, is what determines this topography. These relationships have a bearing on the patient's final results when a surgeon attempts to form an acute cervicomental angle (CMA), shape a distinct inferior mandibular border, or accentuate the anterior border of the sternocleidomastoid muscle (SCM), all of which have been thought to contribute to the attractiveness of the neck (**Fig. 1**).[1,3,4] In addition, the anatomic transition of the neck to the lower third of the face (neck-face interface) is fundamental to the overall facial aesthetic. Classification schemas have been developed by several investigators to characterize the aging process of the face and neck.[1,5,6] When assessing candidacy for possible facial and neck rejuvenation, the senior author uses a 3-tier classification system, which focuses

[a] Meridian Plastic Surgeons, 170 West 106th Street, Indianapolis, IN 46290, USA; [b] Department of Otolaryngology—Head & Neck Surgery, Indiana University School of Medicine, Indianapolis, IN 46202, USA
* Corresponding author. Meridian Plastic Surgeons, 170 West 106th Street, Indianapolis, IN 46290.
E-mail address: sperkins@meridianplastic.com

Facial Plast Surg Clin N Am 22 (2014) 161–170
http://dx.doi.org/10.1016/j.fsc.2014.01.009
1064-7406/14/$ – see front matter © 2014 Elsevier Inc. All rights reserved.

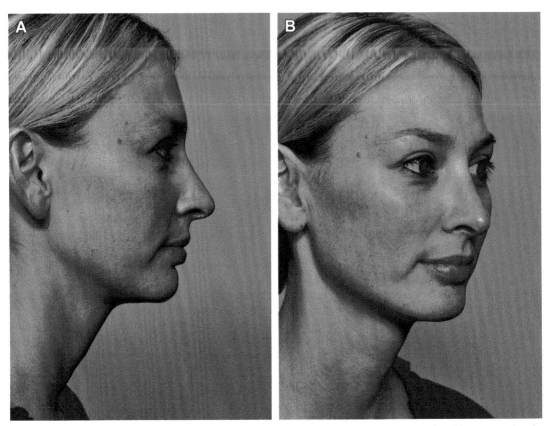

Fig. 1. (*A, B*) A youthful neck with an acute CMA, distinct inferior mandibular border, and visible anterior border of the sternocleidomastoid muscle.

on skin laxity, submental lipoptosis, jowling, platysmal banding, and the CMA.[7]

The neck can be separated into anterior and posterior triangles, and although the posterior neck can show signs of aging, this article focuses on the anterior neck. The anterior triangles of the neck are bounded inferiorly by the sternal notch and clavicles, and laterally by the sternocleidomastoid muscle (SCM) bilaterally. The trachea, thyroid, and cricoid cartilages represent the midline, dividing right from left. Posterior to the SCM demarcates the start of the posterior triangle, with the trapezius, occipital scalp, and cervical vertebrae forming the posterior boundaries. The superior aspect of the anterior neck is delineated by the chin and the lower mandibular line and angle, rising toward the mastoid processes more posteriorly.[3]

Analyzing each layer from superficial to deep, therapies can then be tailored to specific anatomic structures and relationships, further individualizing a patient's treatment plan based on previously agreed-on goals and expectations.

Skin

Skin changes within the neck can often be the most prominent feature seen with aging. Understanding the anatomic and physiologic processes involved with skin aging is of great importance in formulating individual treatment algorithms.

The sensory innervation of the anterolateral neck skin is derived from the transverse cervical nerves (C2, C3, C4) as they sweep across the neck from around the lateral border of the SCM. The arterial blood supply of the superficial anterolateral neck is derived from branches of the subclavian arteries, as well as perforating branches from the external carotid arteries. The intermuscular and superficial fascias serve as the framework for the vessels coursing to the skin. The external jugular vein and anterior communicating veins join the anterior jugular system and travel underneath the platysma to drain the superficial neck structures.[8]

The skin acts as a protective barrier that is continuously in contact with the environment, undergoing not only chronologic aging but also photoaging as a consequence of primarily sun-induced damage from ultraviolet irradiation.[9] Sun-induced skin aging (photoaging), like chronologic aging, is a cumulative process. Both processes lead to the formation of reactive oxygen species and resultant damage to cellular components, including membranes, enzymes, nucleic acids, and proteins, and disruption to the interactions between them.[9,10] Additional processes that result in the clinical appearance of aging include shortening of chromosomal telomeres, hormonal influences, as well as an age-associated decline in anabolic signaling molecules and receptors, and upregulation of the reciprocal catabolic factors.[9,10] These cellular perturbations manifest clinically as xerosis, laxity, wrinkles, droopiness, loss of hair, and loss of color from melanocyte depletion and decreased tyrosinase activity.[10] Poikiloderma of Civatte is a common dermatologic condition seen in aging female patients that can cause cosmetic imperfections in the skin of the neck and chest. Often difficult to clear clinically, patients can show atrophy, pigmentary changes, as well as telangiectasia formation.[11]

On histology, epidermal senescence primarily results in a decrease in the number of melanocytes and Langerhans cells. In contrast, most clinical aging and histologic changes occur within the dermis, with hypocellularity and flattened dermoepidermal junction rete ridges. There is disintegration of the dermal matrix leading to volume loss, as well as findings of fewer and looser collagen fibers and functional fibroblasts.[10,12] A summaries of the histologic changes accompanying skin aging is shown in **Table 1**.[10]

External factors, such as gravity, play a large role in the clinical appearance of the aging neck when taken in combination with the cellular changes mentioned earlier. The constant force of gravity exerts a mechanical pull on the already unsupported and lax skin. This mechanical pull exposes the changes related to fat depletion, fat accumulation, or herniation, as well as the changes related to loss of structural support from the deeper structures as the skin hangs and follows their contours.

The physiologic changes observed in skin aging affect management. Regardless of the aging process, surgical considerations should be directed at redraping of the skin over the underlying neck structures, which recreates the contour of the neck and CMA. The skin's ability to conform to the new shape depends on the skin's inherent pliability and texture, and often is related to its elastin and collagen content. In the setting of poor-quality or excess skin, excisional techniques are often necessary to allow redraping of the skin.[2,3]

Good candidates for neck rejuvenation are patients who have moderate thickness to their skin, with minimal sun damage, and who have retained some hereditary elasticity to the skin appropriate for their chronologic age.[7] However, some patients with smooth and nonphotodamaged skin may experience premature loss of skin elasticity, and may have an unsatisfactory duration of improvement. In addition, thick-skinned and overweight patients should not expect dramatic long-lasting results of their neck contouring procedures (**Fig. 2**). The increased weight of the tissues, combined with gravitational forces, further limits the length of time in which the soft tissues remain firm and in an upward vector.[7]

Cervical fascia

Superficial cervical fascia The superficial cervical fascia is a thin layer of connective tissue between the dermis and the deep cervical fascia. This fascia covers the platysma muscle, as well as the cutaneous vessels, nerves, and lymphatics. A distinguishing feature is that this layer contains fat, which leads some clinicians to consider it to be a part of the subcutaneous tissue, and not true fascia.[13]

Deep cervical fascia The deep cervical fascia can be divided into 3 distinct layers with the superficial (investing) layer of the deep fascia covering the structures deep to the platysma, including the

Table 1
Histologic features of aging human skin

Epidermis	Dermis	Appendages
Flattened dermoepidermal junction	Atrophy (loss of dermal volume)	Depigmented hair
Variable thickness	Alteration of connective tissue structure	Loss of hair
Variable cell size and shape	Fewer fibroblasts	Conversion of terminal to vellus hair
Occasional nuclear atypia	Fewer mast cells	Abnormal nail plates
Fewer melanocytes	Fewer blood vessels	Fewer glands
Fewer Langerhans cells	Shortened capillary loops and abnormal nerve endings	—

Adapted from Yaar M. Clinical and histological features of intrinsic versus extrinsic skin aging. In: Krutmann J, Gilchrest BA, editors. Skin aging. Berlin: Springer; 2006. p. 9–21; with permission.

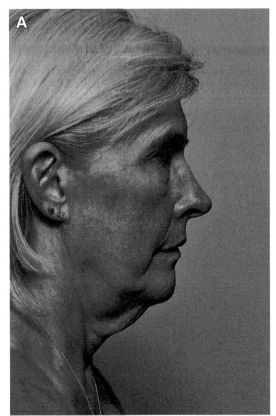
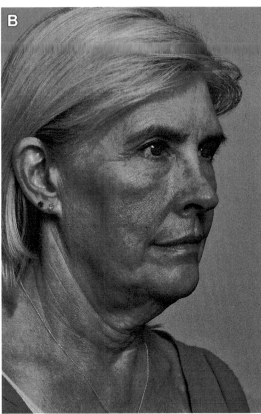

Fig. 2. (*A, B*) An aging neck with changes in the superficial topography (obtuse CMA, loss of a distinct inferior mandibular border, and anterior border of the SCM) with evidence of submental lipoptosis, platysmal banding, and skin laxity. Loss of the delineation of the neck-face interface is also noted with jowling and distinct melolabial folds.

strap musculature, SCM, and trapezius muscles. The submandibular compartments are also enclosed by this fascial layer. The middle or visceral layer of the deep cervical fascia comes around to include the trachea, thyroid, and esophagus, whereas the deep layer envelopes the deep vascular (carotid, internal jugular vein) and neural structures of the neck, and includes the cervical vertebrae and vertebral musculature. Fascial laxity can occur, which is shown by changes in the superficial topography related to descent or exposure of the deep structures, including subplatysmal fat or ptosis of the submandibular glands.

Subcutaneous fat

The subcutaneous fat is found between the skin and the platysma muscle, and is also invested by the superficial cervical fascia. Subcutaneous fat varies in thickness according to the patient's body habitus and weight, and is often a presenting concern for patients. There can be a variable distribution laterally along the surface of the platysma, with patients most often presenting with the largest volume of fat anteromedially. Fat is usually most abundant in the submental area, forming a triangular shape with the apex at the hyoid and base at the mandibular line. Often there is deep extension that is contiguous with the subplatysmal fat at the natural separation of the platysma muscles on their medial aspects.[2] The amount of deep connection in this region depends on the degree of platysmal fibers decussating, which is variable and is discussed later. This fat does not have fibrous connections or septations, making it more easily sculpted through closed or open procedures including liposuction, as well as direct excision.[3]

Within the same subcutaneous plane, patients can develop prominent melolabial folds or jowls descending from the face. Although they are not neck structures, their presence has a significant influence on the perception of a youthful and aesthetically pleasing neck.[3] These structures should be considered in the preoperative analysis and in discussions with the patient, because they can be concomitantly addressed during neck rejuvenation. Most surgical alterations are targeted at reducing the bulk of fat within this area, attempting to develop a more acute CMA and establish an ideal contour. Techniques such as submental liposuction or direct excision are the most common techniques.

Lymphatics

The lymphatic drainage patterns within the neck are complex. Pan and colleagues,[14] using lymphoscintigraphy, eloquently showed the lymphatic channels within the anterior cervical region and isolated 2 distinct layers of lymphatic vessels. The more superficial anterior neck vessels course between the dermis and the platysma, until ultimately penetrating the platysma medially to drain into the submental lymph node basin between the inferior border of the mandible and the thyroid notch.[14] The channels seen draining to the submandibular lymph nodes course from the area just lateral to the platysma border. Deeper channels between the platysma and the deep cervical fascia can be identified draining into the anterior jugular lymph nodes, as well as the supraclavicular lymph nodes.[14]

Superficial muscular aponeurotic system

Within the face, deep to the subcutaneous fat and superficial fascia, is the superficial muscular aponeurotic system (SMAS). Skoog[15] first published descriptions on subfascial rhytidectomy, with Mitz and Peyronie[16] later outlining a distinct anatomic subfascial layer and labeling it as the SMAS.[17] These descriptions have led to the advancement and development of modern facelift techniques, with substantial lasting improvements established by addressing the SMAS layer as it relates to the neck and jawline as well.[18] However, the literature shows significant differences of opinion in the patterns of the SMAS architecture in relation to the face and neck.

In general, the SMAS is 1 continuous and organized fibrous network within the face, contiguous with the platysma muscle as it transitions from the face into the neck.[19] The SMAS is a multidimensional structure consisting of collagen and elastic fibers, fat cells, and muscle fibers.[19] These fibrous extensions course from the periosteum or mimetic musculature through the subcutaneous layers connecting with the dermis. The complex attachments formed allow movement of all the layers as a single unit during rhytidectomy, which holds true for the SMAS junction with the platysma at the neck-face interface (**Fig. 3**). The SMAS extends over the parotid gland laterally, superficial and distinct from the parotidomasseteric fascia. Following the SMAS from lateral to medial there is continuity with the zygomaticus major muscle

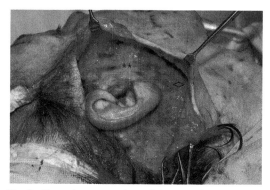

Fig. 3. Clear demonstration of the neck-face interface or junction of the SMAS (**) with the platysma (<>) after elevation and connection of facial and neck subcutaneous dissections.

and levator labii superioris alaeque nasi muscle, but anteriorly the SMAS becomes thin and sparse in the cheek area.[18] There is debate regarding the role of sub-SMAS dissection as a modality in treating the prominent melolabial fold. Histologic studies have shown that, within the medial aspect of the face, there is a zone of fusion among the orbicularis oris, SMAS, and the buccinator muscle at the level of the modiolus.[18,20] During rhytidectomy the SMAS flap is pulled, and the resulting tension is transmitted to the buccinator, orbicularis oris, and modiolus. This technique is associated with a pleasing result at the level of the melolabial fold, with a subsequent lateralization and elevation of the lower third of the melolabial fold and corner of the mouth.[18] Superiorly distinct layers exist between the SMAS and the orbicularis oculi and the temporoparietal fascia, but their discussion is beyond the scope of this article.

Isolating the SMAS and dissecting within the sub-SMAS or deep plane has led to improvements in managing the neck-face interface, midface, and melolabial fold.[6,18,21,22] Additional advantages of the deeper dissection, beyond of aesthetic results and longevity, are related to less subcutaneous dissection and risk of skin flap necrosis.[23,24] However, there are increased risks related to injuring branches of the facial nerve when entering and dissecting within the sub-SMAS (deep) plane.

Aging of the neck secondary to significant jowling, midface descent, and melolabial prominences is common, and procedures addressing the SMAS and the neck-face interface are more appropriate, rather than an isolated neck procedure, which is likely to lead to suboptimal results.[2]

Platysma

The platysma muscle is situated between the superficial and deep cervical fascia, and separates the subcutaneous fat from the deeper structures of the neck. The platysma originates from the superficial fascia overlying the superior aspect of the deltoid and pectoralis major muscle, with insertions at the mandible, depressor anguli oris, risorius, and mentalis muscles superiorly. The platysma is contiguous with the SMAS into the face with innervation from the cervical branch of the facial nerve. The paired, thin muscles course from inferolateral to superomedial, with a variable amount of interdigitation or decussation in the midline submental region. Cardoso de Castro[25,26] further classified the patterns of decussation into 3 types. In type I, which is present in 75% of the population, there is limited decussation of the platysmal fibers, extending only 1 to 2 cm below the mandibular symphysis. Type II is present in 15% of the population, and has the platysma joining completely from the mandibular symphysis throughout the suprahyoid region, essentially behaving as a single muscle. Type III is the least common and is present in 10% of patients, with no decussation of the platysmal fibers at the midline (**Fig. 4**).[2,25,26]

With aging, the platysma begins to lose tone and is pulled laterally, resulting in splaying of the medial fibers. In addition, there is attenuation of the deep retaining ligaments on the medial edge of the muscle contributing to loss of tone. This loss of tone allows the medial edges to descend, leading to development of platysmal bands, which can be exaggerated with contraction. Patients with minimal or no platysmal decussation can have interplatysmal fat in the submental region herniate between the medial edges, which is contiguous with the subplatysmal fat of the deep compartment, further contributing to the appearance of neck aging.[1,2,26]

Aging can result in laxity, redundancy, and banding, which can be addressed with techniques such as submentoplasty or platysmaplasty. The goal is to resuspend and plicate the medial edges, and to excise redundant muscle and fat when necessary.

The deep compartment structures and surrounding neurovascular anatomy are at risk once the plane deep to the platysma is breeched. This anatomy includes branches of the external carotid artery and the jugular venous system as well as the cervical and marginal mandibular nerve branches of the facial nerve. The deeper neck compartment is discussed in detail later.

Subplatysmal deep compartment structures
The subplatysmal compartment (**Fig. 5**) defines the deep plane in neck rejuvenation, and the surgically relevant structures are discussed separately with specific neural and vascular structures mentioned when pertinent to an anatomic region.

Subplatysmal fat With aging, there can be accumulation, depletion, as well as descent of the deep subplatysmal fat. Herniation through the interplatysmal region further contributes to the appearance of submental fullness and an obtuse CMA.

The deep fat can be broken down into the central, medial, and lateral compartments, with Rohrich and Pessa[27] describing compartmentalization by color variations among the fat. The central compartment had a more discrete yellow color, whereas the medial and lateral compartments were pale, similar to buccal fat. The compartments cover the mylohyoid muscles forming a triangular-shaped adipose tissue mass that extends from the lateral third of the mandible to the thyroid cartilage.[27]

When excising fat or liposculpting in this area, the surgeon must exercise caution when resecting centrally, because overaggressive resection may result in a hollow appearance to the neck. The

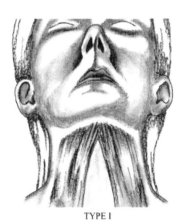
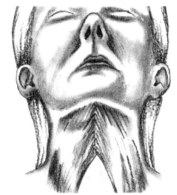
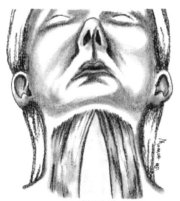

TYPE I   TYPE II   TYPE III

Fig. 4. Anatomic classification of platysmal muscle decussation patterns. (*From* Mejia JD, Nahai FR, Nahai F, et al. Isolated management of the aging neck. Semin Plast Surg 2009;23(4):264–73; with permission.)

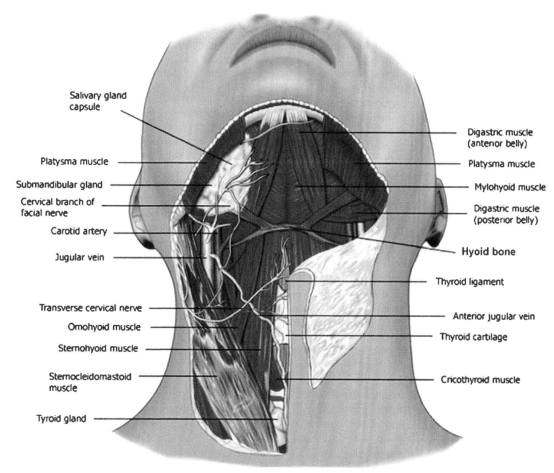

Salivary gland capsule

Platysma muscle

Submandibular gland

Cervical branch of facial nerve

Carotid artery

Jugular vein

Transverse cervical nerve

Omohyoid muscle

Sternohyoid muscle

Sternocleidomastoid muscle

Tyroid gland

Digastric muscle (anterior belly)

Platysma muscle

Mylohyoid muscle

Digastric muscle (posterior belly)

Hyoid bone

Thyroid ligament

Anterior jugular vein

Thyroid cartilage

Cricothyroid muscle

Fig. 5. Anatomic layers and structures of the superficial and deep neck. (*From* Ramirez OM. Advanced considerations determining procedure selection in cervicoplasty. Part one: anatomy and aesthetics. Clin Plast Surg 2008;35(4):679–90, viii; with permission.)

surgeon should always keep in mind that the ideal appearance of the youthful neck maintains a rounded contour as opposed to a more skeletonized appearance.[4] Dissection in this region carries a risk of injury to vascular structures, as well as the cervical and marginal mandibular branches of the facial nerve. In addition, the adipose tissue is well vascularized, with several perforators joining from the adjacent musculature. Vascularized level 1A lymphatic nodes are also encountered during surgical dissection. Fat excision in this region requires bipolar cauterization in order to obtain hemostasis and avoid hematoma formation.

Digastric muscles The digastric muscles consist of 3 distinct parts, with the anterior belly originating from the mandibular fossa, and an intermediate tendon attaching to the body of the hyoid, which then joins the anterior belly with the posterior belly originating from the mastoid notch. The digastric muscles form the boundaries of the

submandibular triangle. Separate nerves innervate the muscle bellies, with the anterior belly being innervated by the mandibular division of the trigeminal nerve via a branch of the nerve to the mylohyoid. An additional branch to the digastric muscle, slung from the facial nerve, innervates the posterior belly. The digastric muscles act to elevate the hyoid and also act as weak depressors of the mandible.

The actions of the digastric muscles on the hyoid are thought to contribute to formation of the CMA, and modifying the muscles for neck rejuvenation and contouring has been under debate, with conflicting practices published.[1,26,28] Some techniques include plicating the muscles in the midline and shaving or excising hypertrophic components of the muscles, whereas others release the suprahyoid tendon aponeurosis connected to the hyoid to deepen the CMA.[1,3] The authors do not advocate maneuvers intended to augment the digastric muscles.

Submandibular glands The submandibular glands are located within the submandibular triangle, which is formed by the digastric muscle bellies with the inferior mandibular edge acting as the superior boundary. The glands are sheathed by the investing (superficial) layer of the deep cervical fascia. The mylohyoid muscle divides the gland into deep and superficial sections, with the deep portions of the gland resting over the hyoglossus muscle. The glands primarily function in the production of saliva, which additionally acts as a carrier for digestive enzymes and immunologic factors.

With aging, patients may develop ptosis or hypertrophy of the glands, with both contributing to contour irregularities in this region. Routine dissection or excision of the glands is controversial because of the inherent risk to the surrounding structures. The marginal mandibular nerve, lingual nerve, hypoglossal nerve, Wharton duct, facial artery, and facial vein are all at risk when manipulating the gland. In addition, neural injury, xerostomia, sialocele, or hematoma formation, possibly resulting in airway compromise, are all complications that surgeons should be aware of when counseling patients regarding partial or total gland resection. Simply suspending the platysma or the fascia overlying the glands to act as a sling can be advantageous in the treatment of ptotic glands without taking on substantial risk, and is the choice of most surgeons. The authors do not encourage the manipulation of the submandibular glands in neck rejuvenation.

SCM The youthful neck is described as having a distinct outline of the anterior SCM border. The anatomy of the SCM defines the lateral boundary of the anterior triangle, which often is the extent of dissection needed in neck rejuvenation. The muscle originates at the manubrium sterni and medial one-third of the clavicle coursing posterosuperiorly to insert on the mastoid process and lateral one-half of the superior nuchal line. The superficial layer of the deep cervical fascia invests the SCM. The muscle is innervated by the spinal accessory nerve, and is involved in turning the head to the opposite side, as well as flexing the head.

Running deep to the platysma and along the lateral aspect of the SCM are the external jugular vein and great auricular nerve (discussed separately). The vein and nerve are separated from the SCM by the investing layer of the deep cervical fascia. This separation becomes surgically relevant when dissecting posterolaterally, because the surgeon should transition to a plane superficial to the fascia of the SCM to ensure that the elevation does not pass deep to the fascia or the SCM. A plane of dissection deep to the fascia could then allow injury to the external jugular vein and greater auricular nerve. The dissection is often difficult posteriorly because of the attenuation of the fat in this area and the stronger dermal attachments of the skin to the fascia and muscle.[17,29]

Great auricular nerve The great auricular nerve is formed by the second and third ventral primary rami of the cervical plexus, and ascends along the SCM to innervate the lobule, the skin behind the auricle, and skin overlying the parotid gland. The great auricular nerve is described as the most commonly injured nerve during rejuvenative procedures of the face and neck, which emphasizes the necessity of having a thorough understanding of its course to avoid injury. As described earlier, it runs parallel to the external jugular vein, crossing the SCM at the junction of the superior third and lower two-thirds of the muscle. This region is referred to as the Erb point, and the nerve divides approximately 6.0 to 6.5 cm inferior to the external auditory meatus into its auricular, mastoid, and facial branches.[1,3,30]

The great auricular nerve can be preserved by exercising the precautions discussed earlier and maintaining a plane of dissection superficial to the fascia overlying the SCM.

Facial nerve The cervical and marginal mandibular nerves are the most frequently encountered branches of the facial nerve during deep dissection within the neck. The cervical branch runs anteroinferiorly from its emergence at the caudal end of the parotid, coursing under the platysma as it innervates the muscle. Disruption of this nerve can lead to lip depressor dysfunction; however, this is rarely clinically relevant, and, if present, full recovery is expected.[31]

The marginal mandibular nerve runs toward the mandibular angle in a subplatysmal plane before turning across the body of the mandible to supply the muscles of the lower lip and chin. The course of the nerve has been described as passing 1.2 to 1.3 cm, or less than 2 finger breadths, below the body of the mandible, with multiple branches encountered in most individuals.[1,3,32] Owsley and Agarwal[33] described anatomic danger zones for the cervical and mandibular branches in a subplatysmal plane. The zone is encompassed by the angle of the mandible laterally, the oral commissure medially, a line 1 cm above and parallel to the mandibular border cephalically, and a line 2 cm below the mandibular border as the caudal boundary (**Fig. 6**).[33] By maintaining deep dissection above the investing cervical fascia the surgeon can protect the branches of the marginal mandibular nerve, with reports of injury ranging from 0.5% to 2.6% during rejuvenative procedures.[3,33]

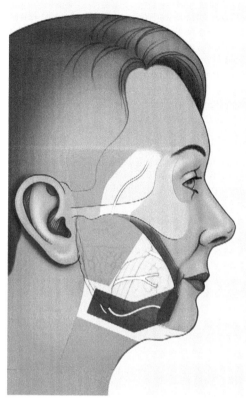

Fig. 6. Danger zones of the facial nerve. Green indicates a safe area, yellow indicates where cautious dissection is required, and red indicates where extreme caution is necessary. (*From* Owsley JQ, Agarwal CA. Safely navigating around the facial nerve in three dimensions. Clin Plast Surg 2008;35(4):469–77, v; with permission.)

Deeper structures

Routine procedures for the aging neck do not commonly violate the visceral (middle) layer or prevetebral (deep) layers of the deep cervical fascia. Further discussion regarding the cervical plexus outflow, lower cranial nerves, internal jugular vein, and carotid artery are beyond the scope of this article. Such discussion is not pertinent to routine procedures for neck rejuvenation.

Mandible As described earlier, the aesthetic appearance and impression of youth can be strongly influenced by the superficial topography of the mandible. Ramirez[3] describes several mandibular landmarks as potential areas that highlight the aging process, including the lateral projection and vertical length of the mandible; the definition and sharpness of the mandibular angle and inferior border; as well as the prominence, height, and width of the mentum. The aging neck can be influenced by changes in mandibular contours seen with jowling, fat descent, submental fullness, or bony atrophy. These changes all culminate

as loss of mandibular definition, which carries implications for the superficial topography of the neck, and potentially for the CMA. In addition, a recessed or atrophic mandible alters the point of transition from the horizontal submental plane to the vertical plane of the neck and affects the CMA. Mandibular augmentation can consequently have a serious impact on the appearance and harmony of the neck and face, as described earlier as the neck-face interface.

Hyoid The hyoid and its relationship to the above-mentioned muscular, bony, and fascial attachments take on a critical role in establishing the CMA. The hyoid bone typically lies at the level of the third cervical vertebrae and this position relative to the mandible corresponds with the CMA.[1] A low anterior hyoid results in the appearance of an obtuse CMA, and the outcomes after rejuvenation are often suboptimal because of its low anatomic position. The ideal hyoid position needed to achieve an acute CMA is posterior and superior. Surgical manipulation of the hyoid is not a routine practice in correction of the aging neck.

Cartilaginous structures

Below the hyoid bone is the thyroid cartilage. Its most anterior projection, the laryngeal prominence, can be seen on inspection of the neck in most men and in some female patients. This prominence was described by Ellenbogen and Karlin[4] as a sign of a youthful neck; however, aggressive dissection in the neck can lead to skeletonization of this structure and may result in unwanted masculinization. The surgeon must be careful when manipulating the structures overlying this compartment. Cartilaginous structures, such as the cricoid or the superior and inferior horns of the thyroid cartilage, are not visible under most circumstances.

Radiographic imaging

Radiographic imaging is not routinely performed in the clinical work-up of the aging neck. In the setting of previous trauma, or for patients with a history of nonaesthetic surgical intervention in the cervical region, considerations for radiographic imaging may be given. Computed tomography or magnetic resonance imaging could be performed for surgical planning. The authors do not customarily obtain imaging in the setting of neck rejuvenation.

SUMMARY

There are a multitude of techniques designed to address the clinical consequences of aging within the neck. Neck rejuvenation and contouring procedures are challenging and continually advancing. Although the techniques are evolving, the anatomy is constant, and surgeons with a firm understanding of the anatomic relationships within the neck are able to deliver consistent and aesthetically pleasing results for their patients.

REFERENCES

1. Caplin DA, Perlyn CA. Rejuvenation of the aging neck: current principles, techniques, and newer modifications. Facial Plast Surg Clin North Am 2009;17(4):589–601, vi–vii.
2. Mejia JD, Nahai FR, Nahai F, et al. Isolated management of the aging neck. Semin Plast Surg 2009; 23(4):264–73.
3. Ramirez OM. Advanced considerations determining procedure selection in cervicoplasty. Part one: anatomy and aesthetics. Clin Plast Surg 2008; 35(4):679–90, viii.
4. Ellenbogen R, Karlin JV. Visual criteria for success in restoring the youthful neck. Plast Reconstr Surg 1980;66(6):826–37.
5. Dedo DD. "How I do it"–plastic surgery. Practical suggestions on facial plastic surgery. A preoperative classification of the neck for cervicofacial rhytidectomy. Laryngoscope 1980;90(11 Pt 1):1894–6.
6. Baker DC. Lateral SMASectomy, plication and short scar facelifts: indications and techniques. Clin Plast Surg 2008;35(4):533–50, vi.
7. Perkins SW, Naderi S. Rhytidectomy. In: Papel I, editor. Facial plastic and reconstructive surgery. New York: Thieme; 2009. p. 207–25.
8. Hurwitz DJ, Rabson JA, Futrell JW. The anatomic basis for the platysma skin flap. Plast Reconstr Surg 1983;72(3):302–14.
9. Fisher GJ, Kang S, Varani J, et al. Mechanisms of photoaging and chronological skin aging. Arch Dermatol 2002;138(11):1462–70.
10. Yaar M. Clinical and histological features of intrinsic versus extrinsic skin aging. In: Krutmann J, Gilchrest BA, editors. Skin aging. Berlin: Springer; 2006. p. 9–21.
11. Behroozan DS, Goldberg LH, Glaich AS, et al. Fractional photothermolysis for treatment of poikiloderma of Civatte. Dermatol Surg 2006;32(2):298–301.
12. West MD. The cellular and molecular biology of skin aging. Arch Dermatol 1994;130(1):87–95.
13. Gadre AK, Gadre KC. Infections of the deep spaces of the neck. In: Johnson JT, Bailey BJ, editors. Head and neck surgery - Otolaryngology. 4th edition. Philadelphia: Lippincott Williams & Wilkins; 2006. p. 665–82.
14. Pan WR, Le Roux CM, Briggs CA. Variations in the lymphatic drainage pattern of the head and neck: further anatomic studies and clinical implications. Plast Reconstr Surg 2011;127(2):611–20.
15. Skoog T. Plastic surgery: the aging face. In: Skoog T, editor. Plastic surgery: new methods and refinements. Philadelphia: WB Saunders; 1974. p. 300–30.
16. Mitz V, Peyronie M. The superficial musculo-aponeurotic system (SMAS) in the parotid and cheek area. Plast Reconstr Surg 1990;86:53–61.
17. Perkins SW, Patel AB. Extended superficial muscular aponeurotic system rhytidectomy: a graded approach. Facial Plast Surg Clin North Am 2009; 17(4):575–87, vi.
18. Gassner HG, Rafii A, Young A, et al. Surgical anatomy of the face: implications for modern face-lift techniques. Arch Facial Plast Surg 2008; 10(1):9–19.
19. Ghassemi A, Prescher A, Riediger D, et al. Anatomy of the SMAS revisited. Aesthetic Plast Surg 2003; 27(4):258–64.
20. Gasser RF. The development of the facial muscles in man. Ann Otol Rhinol Laryngol 1967;76(1):37–56.
21. Hamra ST. The tri-plane face lift dissection. Ann Plast Surg 1984;12(3):268–74.
22. Kamer FM. One hundred consecutive deep plane face-lifts. Arch Otolaryngol Head Neck Surg 1996; 122(1):17–22.
23. Jacono AA, Parikh SS. The minimal access deep plane extended vertical facelift. Aesthet Surg J 2011;31(8):874–90.
24. Parikh SS, Jacono AA. Deep-plane face-lift as an alternative in the smoking patient. Arch Facial Plast Surg 2011;13(4):283–5.
25. de Castro CC. The anatomy of the platysma muscle. Plast Reconstr Surg 1980;66(5):680–3.
26. De Castro CC. Anatomy of the neck and procedure selection. Clin Plast Surg 2008;35(4):625–42, vii.
27. Rohrich RJ, Pessa JE. The subplatysmal supramylohyoid fat. Plast Reconstr Surg 2010;126(2): 589–95.
28. Baker DC. Face lift with submandibular gland and digastric muscle resection: radical neck rhytidectomy. Aesthet Surg J 2006;26(1):85–92.
29. McCollough EG, Perkins S, Thomas JR. Facelift: panel discussion, controversies, and techniques. Facial Plast Surg Clin North Am 2012;20(3):279–325.
30. Alberti PW. The greater auricular nerve. Donor for facial nerve grafts: a note on its topographical anatomy. Arch Otolaryngol 1962;76:422–4.
31. Daane SP, Owsley JQ. Incidence of cervical branch injury with "marginal mandibular nerve pseudoparalysis" in patients undergoing face lift. Plast Reconstr Surg 2003;111(7):2414–8.
32. Woltmann M, Faveri R, Sgrott EA. Anatomosurgical study of the marginal mandibular branch of the facial nerve for submandibular surgical approach. Braz Dent J 2006;17(1):71–4.
33. Owsley JQ, Agarwal CA. Safely navigating around the facial nerve in three dimensions. Clin Plast Surg 2008;35(4):469–77, v.

Preoperative Evaluation of the Aging Neck Patient

J. Regan Thomas, MD[a], Tatiana K. Dixon, MD[b],*

KEYWORDS

• Cervical angle • Hyoid position • Mentum • Platysma laxity • Jowl laxity

KEY POINTS

- Preoperative evaluation of the aging neck patient determines the type of rejuvenation that will be required and the degree of improvement attainable.
- Key anatomic components that should be evaluated are the condition of the skin, amount of soft adipose tissue, mandibular margin, hyoid position, and status of the platysmal muscle layer.
- Chin augmentation in conjunction with other submental plastic procedures can profoundly help improve the overall cervical facial appearance.
- To maximize patient safety and successful wound healing in this elective procedure, it is imperative to consider systemic or complicating medical factors such as whether the patient is a diabetic, on blood thinners, or a smoker.

INTRODUCTION

Facial rejuvenation procedures are of increasing interest to the public. The neck and submental regions are of particular concern to the perspective patient in that both aesthetic and anatomic variations as well as aging changes are easily identifiable and not readily camouflaged. Facelift surgery and the multiple surgical variations of that procedure, as well numerous nonsurgical treatments, are frequent objectives of many aesthetic patients. Successful results of these procedures and treatments depend heavily on appropriate preoperative evaluation and thus, appropriate patient selection, surgical planning, and technique utilization.

Growing general acceptance and popularity of these treatments and procedures have been due to enhanced safety and results, which are in turn related to appropriate preoperative evaluation.[1,2] It has been suggested that when analyzing the face or neck, it may be easier to describe what detracts from beauty rather than what is beautiful.[3] Cervical and neck appearance must display traits associated with youthfulness in order to be typically seen as beautiful. From the time of the early Greeks, proportions and relationships have been described to help analyze the most aesthetic appearance of the face and neck. Back then, a smooth neck was seen by most as aesthetically attractive. Various classifications have been suggested to help identify and categorize neck appearance and potentially assist in developing a treatment plan. These categories or classes usually range from a youthful smooth neck appearance through increments of skin laxity, platysma banding, fat accumulation, chin projection, hyoid bone position, and cervicomental angle.[1,6]

Financial Disclosures: The authors have no disclosures.
[a] Department of Otolaryngology—Head and Neck Surgery, University of Illinois at Chicago, 1855 West Taylor, Suite 2.42, Chicago, IL 60611, USA; [b] Facial Plastic & Reconstructive Surgery/General Otolaryngology, Department of Otolaryngology—Head and Neck Surgery, University of Illinois at Chicago, 1855 West Taylor, Suite 2.42, Chicago, IL 60611, USA
* Corresponding author.
E-mail address: tfeuer1@uic.edu

Facial Plast Surg Clin N Am 22 (2014) 171–176
http://dx.doi.org/10.1016/j.fsc.2014.01.004

The appearance overall of the aging neck is a complex combination of several anatomic structures. The appearance of the skin of the neck often provides insight into the patient's aging process.[6] Both structural and functional changes occur in the skin with aging. Key factors include the intrinsic changes related to aging itself and the degree of photoaging from concomitant chronic ultraviolet light exposure. The typical aesthetic observations include dyspigmentation, laxity, wrinkling, telangiectasias, and a leathery appearance.[7]

Ultimately collagen becomes stiff and is less elastic with the clinical signs of wrinkles and laxity becoming evident in the patient desiring neck rejuvenation. The most successful results in the aging neck patient are typically in patients in whom the aging process has been less severe, who have favorable mandible chin projection, a higher hyoid anatomic position, and are minimally obese. Changes in neck appearance over time are typically the result of multiple factors including UV exposure and damage, genetic predisposition, and tissue aging alterations.[8,9] Chronologic age is an unreliable determinant in that these factors impact the patient's anatomy and appearance over a wide spectrum of time (**Figs. 1** and **2**). The wise and experienced surgeon also utilizes an insightful physiologic evaluation of the patient. This should incorporate the patient's expectations and potential for acceptance of realistic results prior to accepting him or her for treatment.

SURGICAL CANDIDATE SELECTION

Ideal characteristics for surgical improvement in the neck region from an anatomic standpoint more often will be encountered in the healthy female patient. In general, men are often poor candidates because of heavier, thicker hair-bearing skin and soft tissue.

Remnants of normal elasticity within the skin, coupled with a lack of actinic solar and environmental skin damage, enhance the potential results. The obese patient with heavy deposits of adipose fat along the jaw line near the submental cervical area becomes a less favorable candidate as the magnitude of adipose content increases.

A high cervical angle with high positioning of the hyoid and thyroid complex makes a significant contribution to optimum results in the submandibular and neck region. A strong, appropriately projecting mandible and chin configuration increases the likelihood of good neckline appearance results. Surgical chin augmentation and implantation may at times be useful to accomplish that goal. The chin must fit in proportion to the rest of the face on patient evaluation. The patient with poor chin projection appears to have an obtuse, cervical mental angle and a fuller neck appearance. Chin augmentation in those individuals makes the cervical mental angle more acute, the neck better defined, and it creates a better-proportioned face.[10] Relative anatomic issues including some submaxillary gland ptosis may impact results and should also be considered preoperatively.

Other general and systemic considerations are an important part of the preoperative evaluation in the aging neck patient. Ideal candidates have no systemic or complicating factors related to their healing ability or safety during elective surgical procedures. Anticoagulant medications including aspirin and nonsteroidal anti-inflammatory drugs (NSAIDs) should be stopped. Smoking or other nicotine use should be discontinued and arbitrarily avoided at least 3 to 6 months prior to surgery (**Box 1**).[11,12]

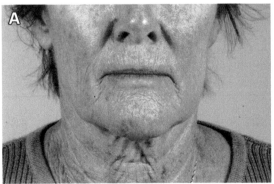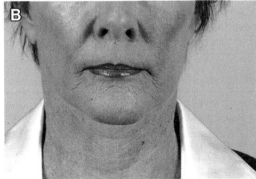

Fig. 1. (*A*) Typical aging face in the pretreatment state with rhytids and skin laxity, jowl formation, and platysmal banding. (*B*) Patient's appearance 1 year following surgical neck correction.

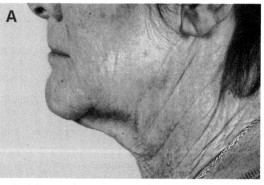
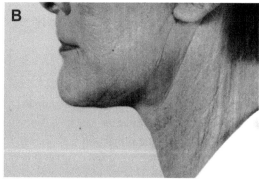

Fig. 2. (*A*) Lateral appearance of preoperative patient with large submental and mandibular laxity in skin and platysmal musculature. (*B*) Patient's appearance 1 year following surgical neck correction.

The ideal patient is identified by the pretreatment evaluation would include the following:

1. A healthy individual without systemic disease
2. Anatomic changes including redundant or excessive skin or ptotic musculature to a degree that significant improvement will be achieved
3. Normal mandibular projection with a high-positioned hyoid, thyroid cartilage complex
4. Superiorly positioned submandibular glands without a ptotic appearance
5. A psychologically stable patient with realistic expectations and goals

Box 1
The ideal patient for preoperative evaluation

1. A healthy individual without systemic disease
2. Ptotic and loose skin and musculature of the neck to a degree to show impressionable improvement
3. Normal mandibular projection with a high position hyoid–thyroid cartilage complex
4. Superiorly positioned submandibular glands without a ptotic appearance
5. Psychologically stable patient with realistic expectations and goals

CLINICAL NECK PROCEDURE EVALUATION
History

The initial consultation and history component is a key pragmatic part of the patient evaluation in potential selection for surgery or treatment. Important elements include the patient's goals for correction and previous history of other related procedures. As noted previously, a thorough history of medical and psychological conditions, medications (with specific attention to anticoagulants including aspirin and NSAIDs), and smoking or nicotine use is imperative.

Physical Examination

Ideally the patient should be positioned in an upright, comfortable examination chair. Appropriate, full lighting should be available. It is often helpful to have a mirror available so the patient may point out areas of specific concern. Likewise, there are key anatomic aspects that may be demonstrated to the patient by the surgeon. Typically, a complete facial examination is completed and discussed even if the neck and submental area is the primary focus of attention and concern.

The examination in the submental and neck region begins with assessment of neck skin quality and elasticity. A head-up and head-down position assessment is useful. The degree and amount of loose and hanging skin and platysmal muscle are identified and quantified including documentation of platysmal bands. The degree and amount of submental fat accumulation are determined by observation and palpation. Columnar neck length is assessed, and the key aspect of the hyoid–thyroid cartilage complex is

---

Box 2
Physical examination elements for the neck

1. Neck skin quality and elasticity
2. Platysmal banding and laxity
3. Amount and location of submental fat
4. Position of hyoid–thyroid cartilage complex
5. Submaxillary gland position
6. Mandibular/mentum projection

Box 3
Characteristics of the youthful neck

1. Well-defined mandibular border from mentum to angle of the mandible
2. No jowl formation
3. High hyoid position with subhyoid depression
4. Cervical mental angle between 105° and 120°
5. Visible thyroid cartilage
6. Visible anterior boarder of the sternocleidomastoid muscle

---

identified and noted, as is the potential cervical mental angle.

The mandibular margin and the jowl formation are noted. Although significant jowl correction is specifically related to facial procedures rather than neck correction alone, often some aspects of fullness from fat accumulation can be improved through liposuction in conjunction with submental liposuction. Ptotic submaxillary glands visible below the mandibular border are documented, and that aspect is discussed with the patient.

Various degrees of retrognathia or poor chin projection, whether minimal or profound, contribute to

the appearance of aging in the neck region. Ptosis of the chin pad and deepening of the submental crease also accentuate the appearance of the aging process. Chin augmentation in conjunction with other submental plastic procedures can help improve the overall cervical facial appearance (**Boxes 2** and **3**).

Of significant importance to accomplishing aesthetic improvement in the neck is the position of the hyoid bone.[13] The position of the hyoid is a key factor in determining the cervical mental angle, and the position is not altered greatly by the aging process (**Figs. 3–5**).[14]

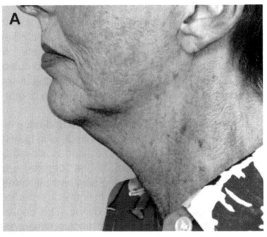
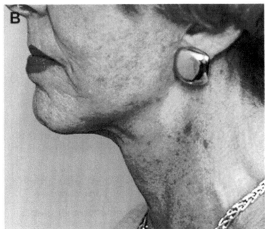

Fig. 3. (*A*) Preoperative patient photograph showing loss of cervical mental angle in the mandibular margin. (*B*) Patient's appearance 2 years following a small chin implant, creation of cervical angle, and correction of mandibular margin.

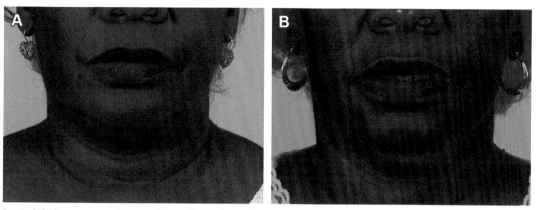

Fig. 4. (A) The preoperative condition of a patient with excess submental fat, skin laxity, and jowl formation. (B) Patient's appearance 1 year following submental liposuction and tightening of the soft tissues.

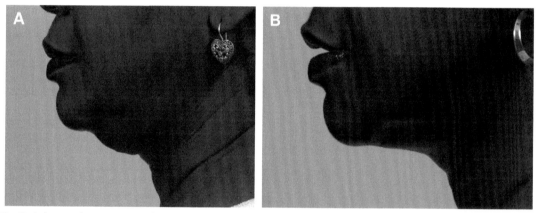

Fig. 5. (A) Lateral appearance of preoperative patient with submental fat and skin laxity. (B) Patient's appearance 1 year following surgical neck correction.

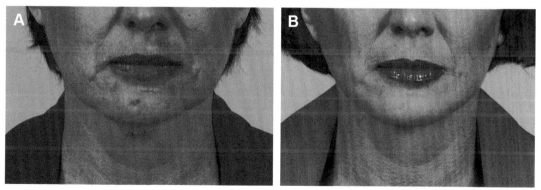

Fig. 6. (A) Preoperative patient photograph showing submental laxity and platysmal banding. (B) Patient's appearance 1 year following surgical neck correction.

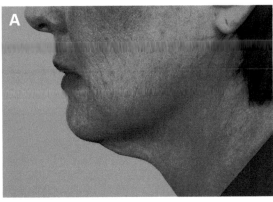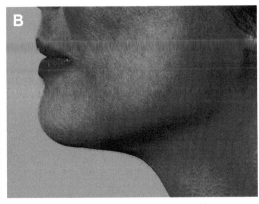

Fig. 7. (A) Lateral appearance of preoperative patient with submental laxity, platysmal banding, and looseness of the mandibular line tissues. (B) Patient's appearance 1 year following surgical neck correction.

SUMMARY

The aging process of the face and neck affects individuals in a variety of fashions. The surgeon realizes that it is a combination of changes in the skin, muscle, fat, and connective tissue producing the characteristics of the aging neck. These characteristics include poor skin tone, changes in skin pigmentation, ptosis of the platysmal muscles, accumulation and grouping of the fat compartments, and facial rhytids. As these are noted through pretreatment evaluation, rejuvenation should encompass each of these findings to achieve results that are satisfactory both to the surgeon and the patient (**Figs. 6** and **7**).

REFERENCES

1. Thomas JR, Humphrey CD. Facelift. Shelton (CT): PMPH-USA, Inc; 2011.
2. Tardy ME, Thomas JR. Facial aesthetic surgery. St Louis (MO): Mosby-Yearbook, Inc; 1995.
3. Lopez MA, Westine JG. Esthetic concepts of the face. In: Thomas JR, editor. Advanced therapy in facial plastic and reconstructive surgery. Shelton (CT): PMPH-USA, Inc; 2010. p. 21–5.
4. Dedo DD. A preoperative classification of the neck for cervicofacialrhytidectomy. Laryngoscope 1980; 90:1894–7.
5. Becker FF, Westine JG, Lopez MA. Direct excision of submental and cervical deformities. In: Thomas JR, editor. Advanced therapy in facial plastic and reconstructive surgery. Shelton (CT): PMPH-USA; 2010. p. 405–12.
6. Burkemper N, Glaser DA. Anatomy and physiology of the skin. In: Thomas JR, editor. Advanced therapy in facial plastic and reconstructive surgery. Shelton (CT): PMPH-USA; 2010. p. 11–20.
7. Rabe JH, Mamelak AJ. Photoaging: mechanisms and repair. J Am Acad Dermatol 2006;55:1–19.
8. Zimbler M, Thomas JR. Pretreatment with botulinum A toxin improves laser resurfacing results: a prospective randomized blinded trail. Arch Facial Plast Surg 2001;3(3):165–9.
9. Larabee WF, Makielski KH, Henderson JL. Surgical anatomy of the face. Philadelphia: Lippincott Williams and Wilkins; 2004.
10. Silver WE, Athre R, DeJoseph LM. Mandibular augmentation. In: Thomas JR, editor. Advanced therapy in facial plastic and reconstructive surgery. Shelton (CT): PMPH-USA; 2010. p. 503–11.
11. McCollough EG, Perkins S, Thomas JR. Facelift discussion, controversies, and techniques. Facial Plast Surg Clin North Am 2012;20(3):279–325.
12. Zimbler M, Kokoska M, Thomas JR. Anatomy and pathophysiology of facial aging. Facial Plast Surg Clin North Am 2001;9(2):179–88.
13. Ellenbogen R, Karliu JV. Visual criteria for success in restoring the youthful neck. Plast Reconstr Surg 1980;66:826.
14. Sandel HD, Perkins SW. Rhytidectomy. In: Thomas JR, editor. Advanced therapy in facial plastic and reconstructive surgery. Shelton (CT): PMPH-USA; 2010. p. 413–28.

A Progressive Approach to Neck Rejuvenation

Mark M. Beaty, MD

KEYWORDS

- Necklift • Facelift • SMAS • Individualized care • Natural results • Facelift evaluation
- Rhytidectomy • Surgical technique

KEY POINTS

- The progressive approach to neck and facial rejuvenation is a comprehensive method for evaluation and correction of common aging changes seen in the lower face and neck.
- The progressive approach takes into account a thorough preoperative assessment but also relies on systematic intraoperative evaluation of each patient as the procedure progresses so as to make surgical decisions based on the maximal amount of information obtainable.
- The ongoing assessments through the surgical procedure itself promote a decision-making process that ensures that appropriate and sufficient steps are taken to correct the aging changes discovered in each patient thoroughly and in a manner most conducive to the structure of their particular anatomy.
- The surgical results with this approach are natural in appearance, as the rejuvenation method chosen is specifically and continuously adjusted for optimal results in the particular patient throughout the evaluation and surgical process.
- The increased burden on the surgeon to master a variety of techniques and to develop the judgment needed to decide in a progressive manner which is the most appropriate for use in each patient is more than compensated for by improved results and greater patient satisfaction.

OVERVIEW AND HISTORY OF RHYTIDECTOMY

Approaches to neck rejuvenation have progressed steadily since the inception of the formal description and teaching of rejuvenation techniques effective in the neck and lower face in the early twentieth century. Beginning with techniques based only on skin elevation and advancement with or without lipectomy, a wide variety of techniques have been advanced and advocated by various groups of surgeons over the years. More aggressive management of the supportive tissues of the face and neck provided increasingly satisfying and durable results but are more complex surgeries, typically with more extended healing times. Most technique development occurred in North America in the twentieth century and is summarized as follows.

Direct Lipectomy

In the early twentieth century, several European surgeons including Lexer,[1] Bourget,[2] and Passot[3] reported successful improvement in the contours of the aging neck and face with techniques involving elevation and advancement of the facial and neck skin. These techniques were associated with various degrees of direct lipectomy. The primary differences among these techniques were length and placement of incisions and the extent of skin undermining performed. At this point in the evolution of rhytidectomy, there was no consideration given to manipulation of the deeper supportive tissues of the face and neck. Results were of limited degree and short duration, with a significant incidence of unfavorable scarring and unnatural appearance due to the tension placed

Beaty Facial Plastic Surgery, 2365 Old Milton Parkway, Suite 400, Alpharetta, GA 30009, USA
E-mail address: mmbeaty@comcast.net

Facial Plast Surg Clin N Am 22 (2014) 177–190
http://dx.doi.org/10.1016/j.fsc.2014.01.001
1064-7406/14/$ – see front matter © 2014 Elsevier Inc. All rights reserved.

facialplastic.theclinics.com

on the skin flap and incisions exceeding the ability of these tissues to support and maintain the repair. Despite these limitations, skin-only rejuvenation procedures were the mainstay of the surgical treatment of neck and facial aging for many decades.

Platysma

The next major innovation in rhytidectomy technique occurred in 1968, with Tord Skoog's[4] description of a procedure that included the platysma muscle in the lower face and neck as a composite unit with the skin flap. This significant improvement allowed much better correction of contours along the jawline, as the inclusion of supportive muscular and fibromuscular tissue allowed a more robust reconstruction of facial contour than was possible with skin-only approaches. The technique was still limited in its ability to manage jowl formation, and the fatty fullness that is often present in the lower face along the jawline was not directly addressed. There was no real consideration of management of the position of midface tissues and the nasolabial fold was not improved significantly. A large series of Skoog rhytidectomies was reported by Lemmon and Hamra[5] and confirmed the limitations inherent to the technique.

SMAS

The next major development in the refinement of rhytidectomy technique was the description of the superficial musculo-aponeurotic system (SMAS) as a discreet fibromuscular tissue layer by Mitz and Peyronie.[6] The recognition that the SMAS comprised the primary supporting and contour-defining structure of the lower face and neck has served as the theoretical basis for most popular rhytidectomy techniques in use today. A variety of approaches to the SMAS and different methods of dissection, manipulation, and repositioning of this tissue have been advocated over time by various investigators. The popularity of different methods and their associated degree of invasiveness has waxed and waned rather than progressed steadily toward more extensive procedures. When SMAS repositioning is limited to the lower face, regardless of method chosen for advancement and fixation, then efficacy for correction of the neck is limited.[3] The mobilization and advancement techniques possible with an SMAS approach allow some choice in advancement vectors for the SMAS, including development of segmented flaps that can advance in differing directions. This may allow greater flexibility of correction in the lower face and neck compared with methods limiting advancement to a single vector. When needed, it is also possible to use different vectors of advancement for the SMAS and the skin. There is a variety of opinion regarding the most favorable vectors for advancement of the SMAS through the range of possibilities from oblique to vertical advancement of the tissue. In recent years, the popularity of more vertical advancements of the SMAS has increased, with advocates arguing that more natural-appearing results are obtained along with better correction of the neck due to the lifting of the platysma as an integral unit with the SMAS along a sliding plane over the deep cervical fascia.

Specific methodology for advancement and fixation of the SMAS covers a wide range of techniques. Plication techniques[7] encompass a group of procedures in which the SMAS is folded upon itself and fixated with suture. The simplest approach to managing the SMAS, the technique is relatively safe with no exposure of the facial nerve. Bunching of the SMAS may occur as it is gathered within the sutures, however, creating the risk of contour irregularities that may be challenging to manage. Imbrication techniques were developed that purported to avoid some of these difficulties. By removing segments of SMAS in a variety of configurations, the necessity of folding tissue can be eliminated; however, the plane of tissue advancement is dictated by the segment excised and may not always provide the optimal improvement in facial contour for a given patient. Additionally, there is some greater risk of the facial nerve being affected when the SMAS is excised, particularly if this excision is done anterior to the parotid gland. In recent years, a variety of named lifts have been advocated, such as the S lift and O lift, which are essentially variations of an SMAS plication lift using specific conformations of suture placement.[8] Thus, the popularity of both plication and imbrication techniques remains high, and in properly selected patients the results are quite good. These techniques are often performed through limited incision approaches, increasing their appeal to patients desiring less-invasive procedures with shorter healing times.

Deep Plane

Hamra's[9,10] description of the deep plane facelift and the composite facelift represent the next major advance in the development of facelift technique. Realizing the limitations imposed by traditional SMAS techniques, including limited mobilization of midfacial structures and minimal improvement at the nasolabial fold, Hamra's techniques advanced a method for mobilizing a robust composite flap of SMAS, platysma, cutaneous tissue, and the malar fat pad. This dissection allows greater mobilization of the midfacial structures and better effacement of the nasolabial fold while preserving blood supply by eliminating multiple planes of dissection over the same area of the face. The deep plane technique is advocated as allowing greater correction of facial laxity through increased tension on the well-supported and vascularized flap that includes SMAS and muscle. It may also offer a safer option for patients having a potentially compromised vascular supply, such as those who smoke or are diabetic. These advantages are in addition to the better result achieved in the midface and nasolabial fold for patients needing correction in this area. The technique itself is surgically more complex and should primarily be reserved for highly experienced surgeons who are used to operating in the vicinity of the facial nerve. Healing time can be variable, with some surgeons believing swelling is more persistent with the deep plane technique and others feeling swelling resolves more quickly. Because the facelift flap is raised as a composite unit, the vector of advancement is in one direction, but the increased tension that can be borne by the composite flap allows for a more vertical lift and more natural-appearing results.

Subperiostial

There have been several descriptions of incorporating subperiostial techniques as a part of facelift technique, primarily described in the midface.[11] This may include midface lift as a stand-alone procedure or may incorporate subperiostial dissection in conjunction with other aspects of a more comprehensive facelift approach. These approaches strive to reposition high-volume tissues, such as the malar mound, to improve facial contour. Especially in light of advances in volume enhancement with both fat and injectable fillers, the popularity of subperiostial lifting approaches has diminished in recent years.

Short Incision

Current demands of patients' social and business schedules have promoted increased interest in procedures using short incisions and incorporating minimal healing time. A variety of short scar lifts have been described including the minimal access cranial suspension (MACS) lift[12] and anterior vertical vector lifts as described by Jacono[13] and Gentile.[3] The focus of these procedures is to apply a more vertical vector to the lifting of the SMAS, which concurrently improves the contour of the neck, often without directly addressing the neck musculature via platysmaplasty.

These techniques can be performed through more limited incisions than more traditional SMAS techniques as well, avoiding extensive skin elevation in the face and often eliminating any skin elevation in the neck. The results of vertical vector lift also have a lower likelihood of creating a pulled or windswept look, as the vector of correction is applied along the lines of actual tissue descent.

Technique Selection

All of the previously discussed techniques have advocates among the community of facial rejuvenation surgeons. During my career, I have been privileged to learn many techniques and approaches to facial rejuvenation through broad experience with various mentors and teachers. Having seen and used most of these methods, the author now recognizes that most of the modern techniques in use for facial rejuvenation are effective and advisable for some patients. There is little evidence for the dogmatic advocacy of a particular technique outside of creating a hook for marketing purposes or because there is a limitation of preferred procedures within the surgeon's personal armamentarium. In fact, now more than ever, the need to match the neck and facial rejuvenation technique chosen to a particular patient's needs is often the most important key to a successful outcome. The algorithm one needs to develop to select the most appropriate technique is complex and challenging, especially when one recognizes that trying to apply any single technique to a variety of patients with differing needs will not yield the best possible outcomes. Choice of rejuvenation method should be guided, but not entirely determined, by the patient's anatomy and extent of aging changes. Especially in the current environment, where many of our patients are active in the workforce, have significant limitations on available recovery time, and/or have no desire to decrease their activity levels, factors other than purely physical evaluation take on increasing importance in the proper selection of technique for each individual.

For all of the reasons mentioned, the development of a progressive approach to neck and facial rejuvenation is desirable for both the physician and the patient. Although this method remains based on a thorough preoperative examination for narrowing the expected parameters of treatment, the final decisions regarding specific technique and the extent of tissue repositioning are made on direct examination intraoperatively. By using a systematic approach to opening incisions and manipulating tissues after evaluating them directly, the degree of intervention is matched more precisely to the needs of the particular patient. This ensures maximal correction of the esthetic problems encountered with the shortest possible incisions and without excessive, unnecessary, or difficult dissection. Minimized healing times increase patient satisfaction, as does the assurance that the needed procedures will be performed through the most limited possible incisions.

TREATMENT GOALS

The overall goal for neck rejuvenation procedures is to contour the neck to provide an aesthetically pleasing cervicomental angle with a smoothly flowing surface that is continuous and consistent with the contours of the lower face.[14] The appearance of excess fatty fullness in the neck should be minimized and bulky or heavy-appearing contours should be eliminated. The skin should be taut, yet free of a stretched appearance and there should be no visible surgical scarring. The skin should follow the contours of the neck and compliment their flow without appearing distorted. There should be no platysmal banding or bulges visible at rest or during animation. It is likewise important to recognize that the neck is anatomically continuous with and aesthetically related to the appearance of the lower face and jawline. Therefore, the neck and lower face must be aesthetically treated as a unit to avoid mismatch in appearance that may be unsightly.

PREOPERATIVE EVALUATION

The preoperative evaluation of candidates for the progressive approach to neck rejuvenation surgery begins with a thorough evaluation of the neck and face with attention to the aesthetic details most related to the final outcome desired in the neck. The contour and position of the platysma muscle serves as the basis for the contour of the neck and as such is the starting point for assessment. Laxity of the platysma contributes to fullness of the neck and effacement of the cervicomental angle due to muscle laxity must be differentiated from excess preplatysmal fat for proper management. Platysmal banding may be observed either at rest or with animation and depending on its severity will dictate either direct management or the possibility of correction by superior and lateral tightening of the platysma. The patient must also be advised of any aspects of his or her neck anatomy that cannot be changed significantly, such as a low-riding hyoid bone.

Fat Assessment

Fatty fullness of the neck is assessed for bulk, aesthetic impact, and location. Preplatysmal fat can generally be managed with suction lipoplasty, whereas bulky subplatysmal fat will require an open approach to the neck with subplatysmal dissection to access the undesirable fatty tissue. Fatty fullness also must be distinguished from contour changes due to platysmal laxity or ptosis of the submandibular glands, as these problems will require additional management to correct, including various sorts of platysmaplasty and consideration of partial resection of the submandibular glands.

Skin Quality and Quantity

Skin quality and quantity are evaluated to assess the likely amount of excision necessary, as well as the ease with which the skin envelope will conform to the underlying reconstituted contours of the neck. Loose, actinically damaged skin will be much less forgiving when trying to develop smooth neck contours than healthy, well-cared-for skin. The placement and likely extent of incisions will depend in large part on the necessary repositioning of the skin. Although incisions can be well camouflaged in the hairline, shorter incisions are desirable from a length-of-recovery standpoint. Reductions in operating time realized with shorter incision approaches are an additional patient benefit.

Lower Face and Jawline

It is also important to recognize the relationship between the lower face and jawline and the appearance of the neck. As people age, it is common to develop descent on the lower facial tissue as the zygomatic and masseteric cutaneous ligaments loosen. This allows some of the lower facial tissue to hang beneath the jawline and descend into the neck, profoundly affecting the contour of the neck. In these instances, it is imperative to correct the position of the lower facial tissues so as to achieve meaningful improvement in the aesthetics of the neck.

There are several classification systems that describe and categorize changes commonly seen in the lower face and neck.[15–19] All attempt to describe the changes seen and associate them with the underlying anatomic cause, thereby giving the surgeon guidance in selection of appropriate procedures for correcting the observed aesthetic problems. Classification systems are useful in facilitating communication about observed facial and neck changes. However, one must exercise caution in placing too much emphasis on a physical examination to determine procedure selection, as many aging changes seen in the face and neck are multifactorial in etiology and may defy specific diagnosis until observed directly at the time of surgery. There are currently no available tools to preoperatively assess the anatomic integrity and tensile strength of deep supportive tissues in the face and neck. Therefore, whereas preoperative evaluation yields a great deal of information for surgical planning, a progressive approach to the procedure itself allows greater accuracy in choosing the best surgical maneuvers for any given individual.

Patient Health

Finally, beyond the anatomic factors influencing the surgeon's choices for specific methods of neck rejuvenation, the preoperative assessment should include evaluation of any health issues, such as tobacco use, diabetes, or collagen vascular disease, which may affect the choice of procedure. Previous facial surgeries or injuries should be thoroughly discussed and assessed for any influence they may have on preferred approach. Additionally, as previously mentioned, the patient's desires for allowable healing time and extent of intervention must be taken into account. Once armed with the full scope of available knowledge regarding the patient's anatomy, health issues, and desires for degree of change, balanced with their available recovery time, the surgeon has the basis to develop an effective, progressive approach to neck and face rejuvenation.

PROCEDURAL APPROACH

After completing appropriate counseling the patient is prepared for surgery. All markings for incisions and landmarks are made in the examining room with the patient sitting up. Proposed incision lines are delineated with surgical marker to the greatest extent deemed likely according to the preoperative examination. Following a progressive approach allows the option of using a shorter incision if the intraoperative observations support such a limited incision approach. The method also requires preparation for the maximal likely intervention so incisions are marked accordingly in both the submental crease and in the periauricular area. Cutaneous landmarks for the anterior border of the sternocleidomastoid muscle, angle of the mandible and course of the frontal branch of the facial nerve are marked if necessary and desired.

Patient Preparation and Anesthesia

The patient is taken to the operating room and placed in supine position. The progressive approach is performed under general anesthesia for maximal control of patient comfort regardless of the ultimate extent of dissection and tissue manipulation undertaken.

Preparation of the face is conducted to the full extent of anticipated dissection and draping is also designed accordingly.

Incision lines are infiltrated with 1% lidocaine with epinephrine. More dilute lidocaine with epinephrine solution is used for a diffuse infiltration of the subcutaneous tissues of the face and neck to the extent they may be undermined. The author does not use tumescent solution because accurate evaluation of the integrity and strength of the SMAS/platysma complex requires that the tissue is not distended.

IV antibiotics and steroids are given.

Platysma Correction

- The neck procedure begins with a small incision in the submental crease. Through this limited access a subcutaneous pocket is created with facelift scissors and advanced for 2 to 3 cm in all directions.

- A Senn retractor is placed and the neck directly assessed for the presence of preplatysmal fat. If significant amounts of preplatysmal fat are encountered suction lipoplasty is performed.

- Pretunnelling of the subcutaneous fatty plane is performed over the entire submental region, limited by the anterior border of the sternocleidomastoid muscle laterally and the thyroid cartilage inferiorly.

- Suction lipoplasty is then performed with appropriate cannulas per the surgeon's preference, clearing the platysma of excess fat. If there is minimal preplatysmal fat present then suction lipoplasty is not necessary. At this point the bellies of the platysma muscle are visible directly.

- Examination is made to evaluate for laxity of the platysma, integrity of the decussated attachment of the medial borders of the platysma, and the presence of platysmal bands. If the problem is limited to mild or moderate laxity of the muscle with a small amount of separation at the medial borders then a midline plication may be performed without further extension of the submental incision. In some cases no further intervention may be needed at all in the submental neck.

- If there is more extensive manipulation needed to correct the shape of the platysma, the incision should be extended as needed up to a total length of 3–4 cm. Through this access the needed modifications to the submental area are made which may include direct lipectomy, division of platysmal bands, transverse division of the muscle, or more extensive platysmaplasty such as the corset technique.

The goal of this portion of the procedure is to create a pleasing cervicomental angle at the level of the hyoid bone and restore a taut submental support for deeper structures including the submental salivary glands. Any platysmal bands are addressed by lysis, excision, corset style oversewing or a combination of the above methods. Additionally, there must be sufficient connection at the medial border of the platysma to allow lift in the vertical direction from the facial portion of the procedure to effectively support the contents of the submental triangle.

Assessment of Skin and Tissue of Lower Face

The next step in the progressive approach is to access and assess the skin and supportive tissue of the lower face. Some information regarding these structures can be determined preoperatively such as skin thickness, degree of photodamage, and extent of observable supportive tissue laxity and deformity. Based upon these factors an initial incision and skin elevation is performed sufficient to access and examine the SMAS to determine thickness, integrity and uniformity of the fibrofatty tissue as well as to assess the skin.

Generally, the initial incision can be limited to the immediate periauricular area extending from the helix of the ear to the lobule using either a pretragal or post-tragal approach as indicated and then coursing up the postauricular sulcus for several centimeters.

A limited skin flap is raised just beneath the dermal plexus of vessels for a distance of only 3 or 4 centimeters. At this point the initial skin and SMAS assessment is made, allowing for performance of a deep plane lift if indicated.

Direct examination of the undersurface of the skin is performed visually and the skin is palpated to assess thickness and compliance.

This examination coupled with information acquired preoperatively regarding any health conditions the patient may have, smoking history and sun exposure history is considered in determining the desirable extent of skin flap elevation.

The author also feels a better assessment of skin compliance is made with a digital exam and physically feeling the stretch present in the skin. This may have a significant bearing on

whether a short flap, long flap, or deep plane composite flap approach is most appropriate for that patient.

Deep Plane Dissection

In many cases there is no need to proceed with a deep plane dissection as the SMAS can be accessed and manipulated with a less aggressive approach; however, if a deep plane approach is selected, the procedure is performed by making an incision through the SMAS along an oblique line two centimeters inferior to the expected course of the frontal branch of the facial nerve as described by Hamra.[11]

- Elevation in the sub-SMAS plane is continued over the masseteric fascia and inferiorly to the mandibular angle.

- This dissection is brought into continuity with a subcutaneous dissection in the midface following the posterior border of the zygomaticus major muscle to protect branches of the facial nerve which enter the muscles of facial expression from beneath.

- The resulting composite flap includes the malar fat pad, dividing the zygomatic cutaneous ligament for complete release of the midface tissues. This creates a robust composite flap capable of supporting thin, tenuous, or damaged skin and allowing maximal effacement of the nasolabial fold and elevation under higher tension of lower facial tissue without increasing tension on the skin closure.

Extensive Skin Undermining

In the author's experience there are also a significant number of patients who have extensive skin laxity in the midface and antero-medial aspect of the lower face who benefit from a much more extensive skin undermining than what is conducted in the standard deep plane approach. Many of these patients still need extended SMAS undermining in the lower face to properly release and correct the jowl and nasolabial fold but, when combined with a long skin flap achieve better results because of:

- Improved skin redraping

- Ability to advance the skin flap along vectors different from the SMAS flap

- An additional dissected plane, which heals and generates new collagen

The specific condition of the skin regarding its laxity and compliance is best assessed when the skin flap is partially raised and this factor makes the progressive approach especially useful in deciding between a deep plane lift and a multiplanar, extended SMAS lift.

Direct Observation of SMAS

Once the initial skin flap is raised and an assessment made of the extent of skin undermining necessary for the patient, the next step in the progressive approach is to directly assess the SMAS for thickness, integrity and compliance. While there are indicators present from the preoperative assessment suggesting the nature of a patient's SMAS such as observed anatomy, history of previous facial surgery, and medical history; the author finds that until direct observation is made the complete combination of factors important for deciding which method of management is best for a particular patient are difficult to discern accurately. During training the author had the opportunity to work with several different facial plastic surgeons, each of whom had a favored technique for managing SMAS advancement. In most cases, the preferred technique was used whether it was the best choice for that particular patient or not. As I gained more personal experience in my own practice, it became apparent that a more systematic, progressive approach would be beneficial to patients. Upon direct observation and palpation of the SMAS the thickness and integrity of this tissue becomes apparent to the surgeon. In some cases it is necessary to incise the SMAS over the periparotid fascia and perform a short SMAS elevation to better visualize and palpate the tissue to complete this important part of the intraoperative assessment.

The key factors in assessing the SMAS are thickness, strength, compliance, and integrity.

- Currently, each of these SMAS assessments is best made by direct observation and manipulation of the tissue both digitally and with instrumentation. Visual evaluation and direct palpation of the SMAS reveals its thickness and amount of fatty tissue present intermingled with the fibromuscular supportive network yielding an indication of likely thickness and strength.

- The surgeon next grasps the SMAS with forceps and mobilizes the tissue layer firmly in all directions. Visual observation and the tactile feel for how the SMAS moves when manipulated in this manner yields an excellent assessment of the inherent strength of the tissue and to what

degree its mobilization affects the fundamental contours of the face. The stretching of the SMAS by forceps manipulation also helps the surgeon to assess the degree of compliance present in the tissue. In the author's experience, tissue of similar thickness and inherent strength may have strikingly differing compliance ranging from a quite inelastic sheet which moves as a single unit to flexible and easily distended tissue which may advance but then stretch back toward its former position as distance from a distal fixation point increases.

- Finally, a thorough visual inspection of the SMAS will reveal whether any tears, scarred areas or thin spots are present. This is most frequently a factor in patients who have previously undergone facial surgery but may be seen as an inherent characteristic, especially in older patients where tissue aging and volume loss may have taken a significant toll on soft tissue integrity.

While the variety of tissue findings is infinitely variable just like the infinite variety of aging changes seen in our patients themselves, the most common findings in assessment of the SMAS are summarized in **Table 1**.

SMAS Techniques

Thick strong SMAS tissue
Thick strong SMAS tissue with good mobility, average compliance and no evidence of weak points or tears is managed with a SMAS imbrication technique, often with an extended sub-SMAS dissection.

- An incision is made through the SMAS in a curvilinear manner over the periparotid fascia coursing from the inferior aspect of the earlobe toward the lateral canthus, terminating just prior to the inferior border of the orbicularis oculi.

- A sub-SMAS elevation is performed to the anterior border of the parotid gland at which time a trial mobilization of the flap is conducted and

Table 1		
Evaluation and treatment of SMAS		
SMAS Thickness	**SMAS Strength**	**Technique Used**
Thick	Strong	Extended SMAS flap
Thin	Strong	SMAS imbrications
Thick	Weak	SMAS plication
Thin	Weak	Multiple SMAS plication

the degree of correction in the neck and lower face observed. As the midline platysma has already been corrected as needed during the first portion of the progressive technique and the platysma extends to interdigitate with the SMAS in the lower face,[20] this mobilization clearly shows the amount of neck correction which will be achieved.

- If the correction of neck, jowl, and lower facial contour is judged sufficient, no further dissection is needed.

- If there is further improvement desired, sub SMAS dissection may continue over the masseteric fascia with facelift scissors, spreading parallel to the course of the facial nerve. This dissection may be carried to the posterior border of the zygomaticus major muscle as needed to achieve the desired amount of contour change in the lower face.

- Once the sub SMAS elevation is completed, the flap is manipulated with Brown Adson forceps or Allis clamps to determine the most favorable vector of advancement. This will usually be in a primarily vertical direction.

- It is often useful to create a small posterior flap by dividing the SMAS just beneath the earlobe which can be advanced to the perimastoid area and affixed, helping to sharpen the cervicomental angle.[11]

- Once the supportive tissue is repositioned, the skin is redraped for closure without tension along a series of vectors creating the most favorable adherence of skin contour to underlying facial contour. The excess skin is tailored appropriately and meticulous closure in layers performed.

Thin strong SMAS tissue

Thin strong SMAS tissue with average compliance is best managed by SMAS imbrication without significant dissection. When examination reveals the SMAS layer having good strength but less than average thickness, the likelihood of difficulty elevating the flap increases, particularly posing problems such as tearing or excessive thinning of the SMAS during dissection, reducing the strength of the advancement and repair. Using the progressive approach, the author will opt in this situation to perform a SMAS imbrication with minimal to no extension of SMAS flap elevation.

- A strip of fibrofatty tissue is excised with facelift scissors over the periparotid fascia coursing from the anterior border of the sternocleidomastoid muscle around the lobule and then in an "S" shaped course toward the lateral canthus

- A minimal elevation of the SMAS flap may be conducted, if indicated.

- The flap is then advanced in a primarily vertical vector, closing the edges of the SMAS excision onto each other meticulously. This allows maximal directed advancement of the supportive facial structures without bunching of tissue. There is opportunity to adjust the amount of advancement during the procedure by further trimming the edges of the SMAS excision or by incorporating a slight overlap of tissue in the SMAS closure.

The healing process for the imbricated SMAS yields a sturdy closure with a completely reconstructed fibrofatty tissue unit which is not reliant on long-term suture retention. Like the extended SMAS elevation technique, the SMAS imbrication technique allows advancement of the skin along a vector which may differ from that used to advance the SMAS, increasing the flexibility of options available to the surgeon for skin contouring during closure.

Thick weak SMAS tissue

Thick but weak and fatty SMAS tissue, whether demonstrating previous tears or not, is managed by SMAS plication techniques. In some cases the SMAS appears robust to visual examination but when manipulated proves to be quite fatty and easily torn. Manipulation in multiple vectors will reveal poor contour correction with advancement of the fibrofatty tissue as the inherent weakness and tendency to tear precludes the establishment of adequate support by repositioning of the tissue as a unit. In this instance, the progressive approach to neck and face lifting entails using a SMAS plication technique. The primary advantage of plication maneuvers in this setting is that the SMAS is supported by placement of permanent suture to gather tissue together rather than relying on the inherent strength of the tissue itself to support the facial contour changes. There are many techniques for SMAS plication described, including but not limited to the S-lift, O-lift, minimal access cranial suspension (MACS) lift, and Quicklift.[8,12,21] Plication lifts all achieve their effect by gathering facial tissues upon themselves with gathering or folding sutures. The repositioning of tissues can be accomplished in multiple vectors depending on the specific placement of the sutures used. An additional potential advantage of plication techniques is that tissue gathered into the midface area may have a volumizing effect, further enhancing the overall contours of the neck and face.

Like all aspects of the progressive approach to neck and facial rejuvenation, selection of the specific suture placement for the SMAS plication is dependent upon the needs of the particular patient. While a primarily vertical vector is generally preferred, there may be aesthetic advantages to creating some oblique component to tissue advancement in certain patients. Rather than rigidly adhering to one approach, (phrase deleted) selection of the best placement of plication sutures can be made intraoperatively as the contour changes observed with differing amounts and vectors of tissue movement are directly assessed as the surgeon manipulates the tissue. Depending on the specific situation, either standard or self-retaining barbed sutures may be used. Patterns of suturing may range widely, with various patterns of purse-string suture, running linear closures or interrupted mattress or figure of eight sutures all having potential efficacy, depending on the patient's needs. Again, the specific pattern depends upon the direction of advancement desired and the quality and nature of the tissue encountered. Once the SMAS is advanced, skin tailoring is undertaken. Incisions are kept as short as practical while allowing smooth and complete redraping of the skin, however, extension of incisions is performed as needed along previously marked extended incision lines to prevent dog ears or tension on the closure.

Thin weak SMAS tissue

Thin and weak SMAS tissue is generally managed by plication techniques using multiple plication points. Gathering of large areas of SMAS tissue may not be practical in this group of patients. Accurate advancement along the desired vectors of correction is best achieved in these patients by placing multiple, interrupted mattress or figure of eight sutures to individually correct a series of contiguous but limited areas, thereby avoiding distortions that may occur by trying to broadly gather a weak or tenuous SMAS layer into larger plicated folds. The author generally proceeds sequentially from superior to inferior in placing the plication sutures, adjusting the vector of each as needed to best repair the weakness in the SMAS at that particular point. Once the desired contours are achieved, the tissue is examined for any excessive lumping or irregularity, which can be corrected by replacing the offending sutures or by trimming areas of gathered SMAS tissue selectively. As with all plication techniques, the dissection plane containing the facial nerve is not approached, increasing safety when compared to a potentially

difficult sub-SMAS dissection when the tissue is weak, thin, and easily torn. Skin flap tailoring and incision closure is performed as previously described for other procedural options.

COMPLICATIONS

Neck and facelift complications are well-recognized and those most frequently cited are primarily composed of unfavorable scarring, hematoma, seroma, and motor nerve damage. Although not considered complications, an experienced facial rejuvenation surgeon recognizes that undercorrection of aging changes, unnatural appearance, and extended recovery time are extremely distressing to patients, leading to dissatisfaction. Each of these issues is minimized by use of the progressive approach to neck and facial rejuvenation. The approach is designed to ensure that an appropriate, individualized dissection technique will be used for each patient. Limiting dissection and tissue manipulation to only what is necessary for each individual patient decreases the overall risk and incidence of hematoma, seroma, unfavorable scarring, and nerve damage. Objective intraoperative evaluation of the supportive structure of the face ensures adequate correction with natural tissue draping. Because the progressive approach encourages performing only the intervention necessary to correct the patient's concerns, recovery time is kept to a minimum.

POSTOPERATIVE CARE

Postoperative care for patients undergoing the progressive approach to neck and face lifting is explained to the patient and his or her caregiver before the procedure when questions can be thoroughly reviewed and answered. Dressings are applied in the operating room and are generally composed of elastic compression dressings for neck support, lower facial compression, or both. Appropriate bolsters of gauze are placed as well, particularly in the periauricular area. Drains are usually not necessary but may be placed in the neck occasionally, if indicated. The dressing is worn full-time for the first 24 to 48 hours, after which removal for parts of the day is allowed. The patient is instructed in the office on the first postoperative day how to clean the incisions and is allowed to shower and wash the hair with baby shampoo on the second postoperative day. Patients are placed on antibiotics for the first week postoperatively and most are placed on a short course of steroid to minimize swelling. Physical activity is kept to ambulation and light activity around the house for at least the first week. Sutures and clips are removed between 5 and 10 days postoperatively. No heavy lifting or exercise is allowed for the first 2 to 3 weeks postoperatively. Makeup can be applied by the 10th postoperative day and may be helpful for covering bruised areas.

EXPECTED RECOVERY

Most patients are feeling well enough to participate in regular daily activities after the second week following surgery. Depending on the extent of surgery needed and the patient's physiology, there will be variable amounts of swelling and bruising. This will gradually resolve during the recovery phase. Anti-inflammatory preparations, such as arnica montana, can be helpful in many patients for speeding the resolution of swelling and bruising. Overall, most patients can be back to their daily routine by 3 weeks after surgery, or earlier in some cases.

OUTCOMES

The author has incorporated the progressive approach to neck and facial rejuvenation in his practice for the past 3 years. The approach has been used on a wide variety of patients ranging in age from their mid 40s to their mid 60s. A wide range of anatomic corrections have been undertaken, including neck deformities ranging from heavy necks with extensive preplatysmal fat and low hyoid placement to patients with primarily loose skin with platysmal banding. Using the progressive approach, a satisfactory improvement is seen in this wide variety of patients, as seen in the examples that follow. The additional benefits of keeping recovery time, swelling, and bruising to a minimum has increased patient satisfaction

and compliance with postoperative instructions in the author's experience.

- In this example, we see a patient in her late 40s, desiring improvement in neck contour, platysmal banding, and lower facial contour (**Fig. 1**). In this case, exploration of the neck revealed significant platysmal bands that were managed with a midline plication. Lower facial exploration revealed strong but relatively thin fibrofatty tissue. An SMAS imbrication procedure was performed, producing an excellent correction of the neck and jawline, as well as good effacement of the nasolabial folds.

- In the next example, the patient, in her early 50s (**Fig. 2**), demonstrated moderate to severe aging changes of the lower face and neck including heavy platysmal bands, moderate jowling, and significant deepening of the nasolabial folds. Following the progressive approach, she required excision and midline imbrication of her platysmal bands. The patient was found to have a robust SMAS layer, which was managed by dissection of an extended SMAS flap with multivector repositioning. Excellent correction of the neck and lower facial contour was achieved with improvement of the nasolabial folds while retaining a very natural appearance.

- In this example, the patient, in her early 40s (**Fig. 3**), desired a smoother, more taut appearance to the lower face. The neck exploration demonstrated no significant laxity so only minimal suction lipoplasty was performed. A short skin flap was raised and SMAS manipulation revealed an excellent response to direct folding of the tissue. A plication procedure was

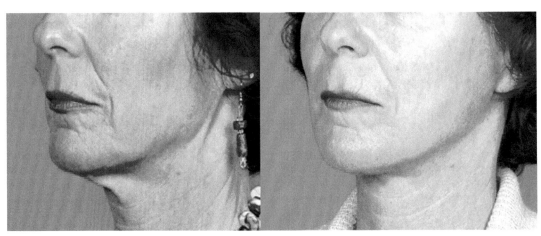

Fig. 1. Patient in her late 40s desiring improvement in neck contour, platysmal banding, and lower facial contour.

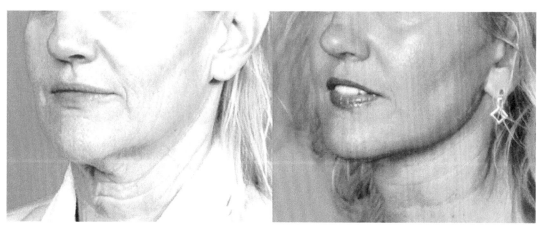

Fig. 2. Patient in her early 50s demonstrating moderate to severe aging changes of the lower face and neck including heavy platysmal bands, moderate jowling, and significant deepening of the nasolabial folds.

performed, advancing tissue in a shaped manner to yield improved tightness of the lower face as well as volumization of the midface.

- This patient, in her early 60s (**Fig. 4**), demonstrated significant laxity and contour deformity of the lower face and neck. Neck exploration showed minimal fat but multiple areas of platysmal banding that were discontinuous. Individual band management with excision of tissue and imbrication was conducted to restore a smooth and strong platysmal sling. The SMAS layer in the lower face was found to be thin with several discontinuous areas on initial examination. A long skin flap was elevated, exposing the SMAS broadly and multiple plications performed to achieve advancement and support without risk of tearing or disrupting the tissue. Good improvement of neck and facial contours was achieved while retaining a natural appearance.

- This patient in her early 50s (**Fig. 5**) wanted improvement of sagging neck and jowls, as well as reduced prominence of the nasolabial folds. She was a former cigarette smoker who had quit in the past year. On elevating an initial skin flap, the subdermal vascular plexus appeared tenuous and a robust SMAS layer noted. The patient was managed with a deep plane facelift achieving her goals of maximal correction of the neck, jawline, and nasolabial fold in a safe manner with minimal risk of skin compromise. The composite deep plane flap allowed enough tension to be placed on the tissue suspension that the neck laxity and platysmal banding were corrected without direct excision or plication.

- This male patient in his early 50s (**Fig. 6**) demonstrates heavy tissue in both the lower face and neck and desired a more refreshed appearance. The neck exploration revealed modest

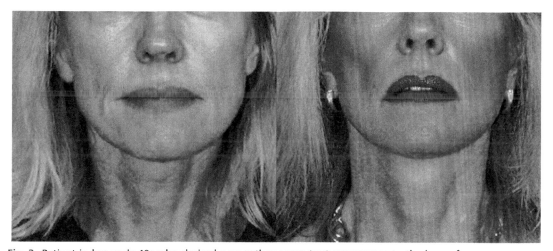

Fig. 3. Patient in her early 40s who desired a smoother, more taut appearance to the lower face.

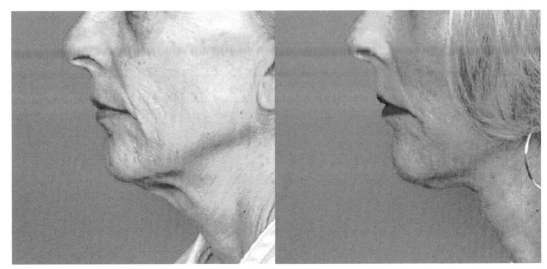

Fig. 4. Patient in her early 60s demonstrating significant laxity and contour deformity of the lower face and neck.

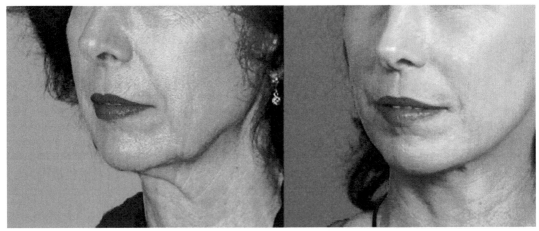

Fig. 5. Patient in her early 50s seeking improvement of sagging neck and jowls, as well as reduced prominence of the nasolabial folds.

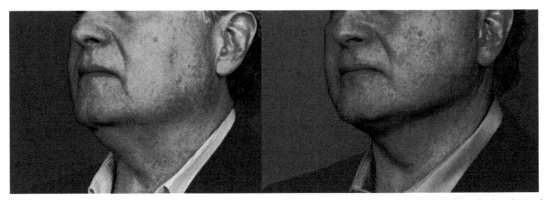

Fig. 6. Male patient in his early 50s demonstrating heavy tissue in both the lower face and neck and who desired a more refreshed appearance.

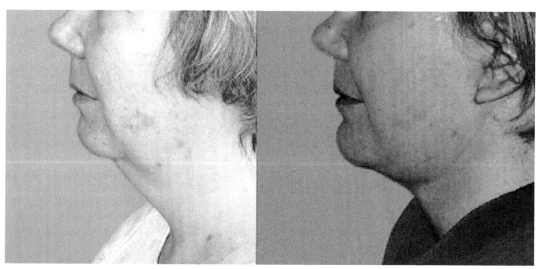

Fig. 7. Female patient in her late 40s with a very heavy neck and extensive jowling that completely obscured her jawline.

preplatysmal fat and significant muscle laxity. Midline platysmal plication corrected the laxity and a combination of suction and direct lipectomy removed the excessive bulk from the neck. An SMAS imbrication lift was performed to manage the lower facial laxity and complete correction of the heavy appearance in the neck while maintaining a natural appearance without overcorrection or feminization of the face.

- This female patient in her late 40s (**Fig. 7**) had a very heavy neck with extensive jowling that completely obscured her jawline. The neck exploration revealed extensive preplatysmal fat and laxity of the muscle. Suction lipoplasty and platysmal plication provided a surprising degree of correction and revealed that while the hyoid bone was modestly low, a nice cervicomental angle could be achieved. An extended SMAS flap dissection provided much improved contour to the jawline while maintaining the fundamental shape and softness of her facial features.

SUMMARY

The progressive approach to neck and facial rejuvenation is a comprehensive method for evaluation and correction of common aging changes seen in the lower face and neck. Rather than focusing on the merits of a particular procedure and developing ways of applying the procedure to patients' needs, this approach first focuses on the patients' needs and then attempts to accurately select and perform the best procedure to address those needs. The progressive approach takes into account a thorough preoperative assessment but also relies on systematic intraoperative evaluation of each patient as the procedure progresses so as to make surgical decisions based on the maximal amount of information obtainable. Using this approach better ensures that incisions and dissection are kept to a minimum, thereby decreasing the likelihood of visible scarring or tissue distortion and reducing recovery times. At the same time, the ongoing assessments through the surgical procedure itself promote a decision-making process that ensures appropriate and sufficient steps are taken to correct the aging changes discovered in each patient thoroughly and in a manner most conducive to the structure of their particular anatomy.

The author's development of this approach represents a gradual evolution of technique over years of practice and was motivated by his dissatisfaction with reliance on a single or primary set of surgical approaches. The author has been fortunate to train with and observe excellent surgeons who used different techniques for management of the aging neck and lower face and therefore has an extensive body of knowledge and experience to draw on. By gaining experience in many surgical techniques, the ability to conduct an accurate and ongoing assessment of the best possible intervention at each step of the treatment process is developed. The surgical results with this approach are natural in appearance, as the rejuvenation method chosen is specifically and continuously adjusted for optimal results in the particular patient throughout the evaluation and surgical process. The additional advantage of minimizing unneeded dissection and tissue manipulation shortens the recovery process, increasing patient satisfaction. The increased burden on the surgeon to master a variety of techniques and to develop the judgment needed to decide in a progressive manner which is the most appropriate for use in each patient is more than compensated for by improved results and greater patient satisfaction.

REFERENCES

1. Lexer E. Die gemsamte Wiederherslellung schiurgie, vol. 2. Leipzig (Germany): JA Barth; 1931.
2. Lam SM. Julien Bourguet: father of cervical thytidectomy. Arch Facial Plast Surg 2004;6(2):137.
3. Gentile RD. Mixed-plane rhytidectomy: the superior vertical-vector approach to rejuvenation of the neck. In: Gentile RD, editor. Neck rejuvenation. New York: Thieme; 2011. p. 56–81.
4. Skoog T. Plastic surgery: new methods and refinements. Philadelphia: WB Saunders; 1974.
5. Lemmon ML, Hamra ST. Skoog thytidectomy: a five-year experience with 577 patients. Plast Reconstr Surg 1980;65(3):283–97.
6. Mitz V, Peyronie M. The superficial musculo-aponeurotic system (SMAS) in the parotid and cheek area. Plast Reconstr Surg 1976;58(1):80–8.
7. Beaty MM. Imbrication, plication, and wide undermining techniques. In: Gentile RD, editor. Neck rejuvenation. New York: Thieme; 2011. p. 82–91.
8. Saylan Z. The S-lift for facial rejuvenation. Int J Cosmet Surg 1999;7:18–22.
9. Hamra ST. The deep-plane rhytidectomy. Plast Reconstr Surg 1990;86(1):53–61.
10. Hamra ST. Composite rhytidectomy. Plast Reconstr Surg 1992;90(1):1–13.
11. Quatella VC, Villano ME. Male rhytidectomy. Facial Plast Surg Clin of North Am. Philadelphia: WB Saunders; 1999.
12. Tonnard P, Verpaele A, Monstrey S, et al. Minimal access cranial suspension lift: a modified S-lift. Plast Reconstr Surg 2002;109(6):2074–86.
13. Jacono AA, Parikh SS. The Minimal Access Deep Plane Extended Vertical Facelift. Aesthetic Surg J 2011;31(8):874–90.
14. Kolstad CK, Sykes JM. Evaluation of the anatomy and aging-related changes of the neck. In: Gentile RD, editor. Neck rejuvenation. Newyork: Thieme; 2011. p. 13–20.
15. Matarasso A, Matarasso SL, Brandt FS, et al. Botulinum A exotoxin for the management of platysmal bands. Plast Reconstr Surg 1999;103(2):645–52.
16. Kamer FM, Letkoff LA. Submental surgery. A graduated approach to the aging neck. Arch Otolaryngol Head Neck Surg 1991;117(1):40–6.
17. Rohrich RJ, Rios JL, Smith PD, et al. Neck rejuvenation revisited. Plast Reconstr Surg 2006;118(5):1251–63.
18. Dedo DD. "How I do it"—plastic surgery. Practical suggestions on facial plastic surgery. A preoperative classification of the neck for cervicofacial rhytidectomy. Laryngoscope 1980;90(11 Pt 1):1894–6.
19. McCullough EG. The McCullough facial rejuvenation system: a condition-specific classification algorithm. Facial Plast Surg 2011;27(1):112–23.
20. Miller PJ, Zoumalan RA, Carron MA. The anatomy and physiology of the neck. In: Gentile RD, editor. Neck rejuvenation. New York: Thieme; 2011. p. 1–12.
21. Brandy DA. The quicklift: a modification of the S lift. Cosm Derm 2004;17(6):351–60.

Noninvasive Treatment of the Neck

Robert W. Brobst, MD[a],*, Maria Ferguson, BS, ME[b],
Stephen W. Perkins, MD[b]

KEYWORDS

- Noninvasive • Neck tightening • Neck lift • Intense focused ultrasound • Ulthera

KEY POINTS

- Intense focused ultrasound is a noninvasive treatment option that can provide clinical results.
- Assessment of patient candidacy is critical but does not guarantee a treatment response.
- Current high-density treatment protocols have not markedly increased reproducibility or objective results in the authors' experience.
- Satisfaction may be related to minimal expectations from a no-downtime treatment modality.
- Patient selection and counseling are paramount, because patients with expectations on par with surgical treatment modalities are disappointed.

 A video of Ulthera treatment accompanies this article at http://www.facialplastic.theclinics.com/

INTRODUCTION

With the ever-growing social acceptance of cosmetic interventions to help patients look and feel their best, facial and neck treatments for the effects of aging and obesity are expanding. The desired areas of improvement are submental lipoptosis, skin laxity, platysmal banding, and jowling. Currently, the gold standard for improvement remains a surgical solution. Submental liposuction, corset submentoplasty, an isolated neck lift, or neck lift in concert with a facelift all provide an immediate, substantial improvement. These surgical treatments, tailored to the individual needs of patients, can offer long-term results at a lower final cost to patients. For many reasons, however, not every patient desires a surgical modality. Finding time in a busy schedule, general operative anxiety, and financial limitations are the authors' patients'

most common reasons given for seeking treatment alternatives.

The alternative, nonsurgical device options are similar in their goals to achieving an improved neckline. Different from the surgical treatment by direct tissue excision and repositioning, the nonsurgical technologies depend on thermal tissue disruption and the healing response to obtain the desired result. In current clinical use, this disruption can be accomplished through a variety of methods, including intense pulsed light, nonablative lasers, and radiofrequency bulk heating. These modalities attempt to preserve the epidermis while creating enough heat in the target tissues. Although protein denaturation begins at approximately 45°C, the goal is to reach greater than 60°C to break the collagen heat sensitive bonds and 65°C for denaturation of collagen and contraction.[1] Most of these

Disclosure Statement: M. Ferguson previously was a part-time Clinical Applications Specialist for Ulthera, Inc. Drs R.W. Brobst and S.W. Perkins have no financial conflicts.
[a] Brobst Facial Plastic Surgery, 4800 Hedgcoxe Road, Suite 250, Plano, TX 75024, USA; [b] Meridian Plastic Surgery Center, 170 West 106th Street, Indianapolis, IN 46290, USA
* Corresponding author.
E-mail address: drbrobst@drbrobst.com

treatment modalities are unable to heat tissue adequately to achieve a collagen response, and ablative laser treatment modalities can only do so with superficial vaporization of the epidermis. Additionally, the ideal depth of surgical treatment of facial skin tightening and rejuvenation is the superficial muscular aponeurotic system (SMAS) or platysma. It is assumed that this depth is also ideal for nonsurgical methods. Each of the noninvasive treatment modalities discussed previously is limited in its ability to accomplishing both these goals.

INTENSE FOCUSED ULTRASOUND

Ultrasound use as a therapeutic modality has grown from its early investigations for neurologic applications in the 1950s.[2,3] In recent decades, high-frequency ultrasound use for the treatment of both benign and malignant solid tumors has expanded. In this form, ultrasound creates thermal injury as well as a cavitation.[4–7] Trials are under way for the use in benign prostate hypertrophy and approval has already been given for an MRI-guided focused ultrasound for uterine fibroid treatment.[8] The use for breast, liver, prostate, and brain cancers is also being studied.[4,5] A nonablative application of ultrasound for targeted drug delivery also shows promise as a future application.[6]

Alternatively, the application for facial rejuvenation utilizes thermal injury alone through intense focused ultrasound. This is accomplished by a shorter pulse duration of 50 to 200 ms, a higher frequency of 4 to 7 MHz, and a decreased energy quantity of 0.5 to 10 J.[7] This technology was commercialized as the Ulthera System (Ulthera, Mesa, Arizona) in 2004 and several preclinical and clinical studies refined the device and supported its ability to create thermal coagulation points (TCPs) at specific tissue depths (**Figs. 1** and **2**).[9–12] Subsequently, a study by Alam and colleagues[13] led to Food and Drug Administration (FDA) approval for a brow lift indication in 2009.[14] Most recently, Kenkel[15] demonstrated improvement in the neck, giving the device an FDA-approved neck lift indication.[16,17]

TREATMENT GOALS AND PLANNED OUTCOMES

The goals of neck rejuvenation with the Ulthera device are to achieve some improvement in the neckline and skin tightness through thoughtful patient selection and increased energy delivery. An ideal patient is usually a younger patient with a robust wound healing response, mild lipoptosis, and

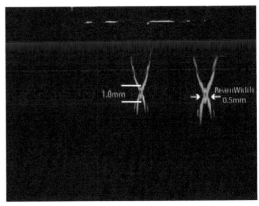

Fig. 1. Schlieren map of intense ultrasound beam profile; 95% of the ultrasound energy is delivered to the targeted, approximately 1.5 mm³, focal point (*bright blue X*). (*From* White WM, Makin IR, Slayton MH, et al. Selective transcutaneous delivery of energy to porcine soft tissues using intense ultrasound. Lasers Surg Med 2008;40:68; with permission.)

good elasticity. An older patient with extensive photoaging, severe skin laxity, marked platysmal banding, and a very heavy neck is not a good candidate. Between these 2 extremes, it becomes even more difficult to predict who will respond; thus, managing expectations becomes paramount. Through a multilayered approach, the authors attempt to see outcomes in good candidates and obtain a response in those who are intermediate candidates through increased TCPs per unit area.

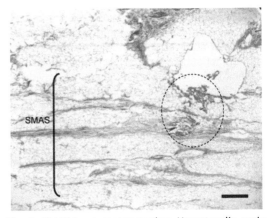

Fig. 2. SMAS treatment targeting. Hematoxylin-eosin staining of preauricular tissue after treatment with intense focused ultrasound. Thermal coagulation point (TCP) identified by the (*dotted circle*). (*From* White WM, Makin IR, Barthe PG, et al. Selective creation of thermal injury zones in the superficial musculoaponeurotic system using intense ultrasound therapy: a new target for noninvasive facial rejuvenation. Arch Facial Plast Surg 2007;9:25; with permission.)

PREPROCEDURE PLANNING AND PREPARATION

With the initial treatment protocols, pain management required the most attention during preprocedure planning. Despite studies reporting minimal or mild pain only (average 3–4 on a 10-point visual analog scale) with topical anesthetic use, the authors' personal findings of patient discomfort were much higher.[7,13] Treatment over osseous structures and repetitive treatment passes elicited the strongest responses, leading to the need of a combination of antiinflammatories, anxiolytics, narcotics, and distraction techniques. Facial field blocks were also offered at patient discretion. Although patient comfort was increased, this led to issues with transportation and the effects of postprocedure facial numbness.

The challenge to achieve desired effects and promote patient comfort led to several Ulthera-sponsored pain control studies, which have been presented, but are, as of yet, unpublished. In these studies, narcotics did not demonstrate any benefit over ibuprofen alone and topical lidocaine did little for analgesia with the 4.5 and 3.0 transducers.[18,19] Most importantly, the company found that lowering the amount of energy transmitted markedly decreased pain levels.[20] Differences in TCP size and split face outcomes could not be identified with the lower transducer settings. Therefore, the newly recommended protocol includes pretreatment with ibuprofen (800 mg) alone and reduced energy settings for each transducer to maximize patient tolerance.

The authors' experience with the new protocol is that, despite lowered energy settings, it remains uncomfortable but bearable for resilient patients. The authors still frequently depend on facial blocks, in addition to ibuprofen and the new settings, for patients to be comfortable during the procedure. Other users have also seen the benefit of facial blocks and local infiltration.[21] This lessens the immediate intensity in most areas with persistent mild to moderate sensitivity noted over the osseous structures. The elimination of narcotics and anxiolytics has made treatment logistics much easier. Overall, additional published studies closely investigating the ideal balance between energy delivery, comfort, and efficacy are necessary.

PATIENT POSITIONING

Patients undergoing Ulthera treatment remain awake and in the supine position during the entirety of the treatment with variable amounts of neck turning and extension during the procedure.

PROCEDURAL APPROACH

An Ulthera treatment of the neck is performed alone or in continuity with a full face treatment (Video 1). Standardized preprocedure digital photographs are obtained after adequately cleaning the face. The patient is then placed in the supine position and the neck is then divided into the desired treatment areas (**Fig. 3**). The thyroid cartilage, inferior mandibular border, clavicles, and preauricular line are marked as landmarks for creation of the treatment areas. Next, each region is marked with a planning card to determine the number of treatment columns necessary to cover the area with minimal overlap (**Fig. 4**). Usually, 5 to 7 columns are possible in the submental/submandibular area and 6 columns are possible below the level of the superior thyroid cartilage. Then, within each column, the measured density is calculated to quantify the number of lines of treatment (**Fig. 5**). These markings then serve as a guide during the procedure.

With the introduction of software updates, use of the device now requires even less decision making and easier calculation of lines. Treatment areas and densities are now automatically recorded in a patient's history. Instead of the default maximum settings, energy density is selected at 1 of 4 preset levels. In the authors' practice, treatment is usually initiated at the second-lowest setting and the energy levels modified based on patient tolerance. Treatment begins at the upper neck region and continues downward as each region is completed in a deep to superficial manner. Ultrasound gel is applied and the handpiece is placed perpendicular to the skin (**Fig. 6**). Correct transducer coupling and verification of depth is confirmed by scanning using the ultrasound images on the monitor. Adjustments should be made prior to treatment to avoid skin striping, incorrect

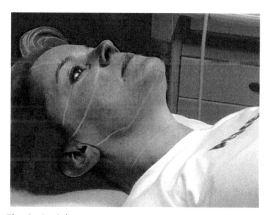

Fig. 3. Facial treatment regions.

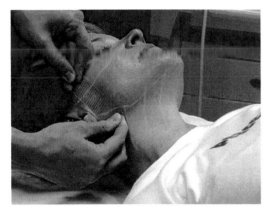

Fig. 4. Marking facial treatment columns with planning card.

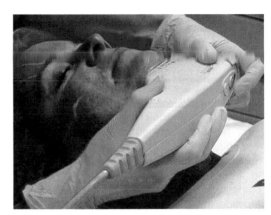

Fig. 6. Ulthera treatment with proper handpiece orientation perpendicular to skin surface. (*Courtesy of* Ulthera, Mesa, AZ; with permission.)

treatment depth, and treatment of inappropriate tissue (major vessels, thyroid tissue, and osseous or cartilaginous structures).[7,13] Typically, treatments are performed at a minimum of 2 depths with 1 pass of a 4- to 4.5-mm (0.9 J/TCP) transducer and then retreating the area with a superficial 7- to 3.0-mm (0.30 J/TCP) transducer. This is in line with current recommended treatment protocols. More commonly, the authors follow the first 2 depths with an advanced treatment protocol using the 10- to 1.5-mm (0.18 J/TCP) transducer for dermal skin tightening (**Fig. 7**). These treatments can be combined with full face treatments or performed in isolation. This multiple-depth treatment protocol is based on previous studies where dual-depth treatments improved subjective outcomes on the upper and midface.[21] The ideal neck treatment protocol is still evolving.[7,13,15,16,21–23]

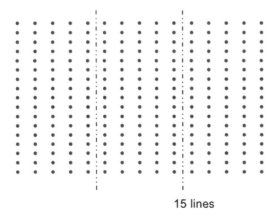

15 lines
3 mm between lines
17 TCPs each, 1.5 mm apart

Fig. 5. Planning card used for line calculation and marking. (*Courtesy of* Ulthera, Mesa, AZ; with permission.)

POTENTIAL COMPLICATIONS

Although the Ulthera device has met all the safety requirements for its use in the face and neck, it is important for novice users to know that complications can and do occur even with this noninvasive device. Usually, 2 to 3 hours of erythema is expected after the procedure, but on occasion this may last up to 1 week or longer.[7,12,13,24] This resolves spontaneously without intervention. Bruising is also an infrequent but self-resolving complication that may be related to transducer selection.[24] Major bruising or hematoma has not been seen in the authors' clinical experience. A complication, largely related to poor user technique, is dermal striping (**Fig. 8**).[7,13] This appears as white wheals or red marks arranged in a linear fashion. It is a result of poor skin coupling, which leads to excessive energy delivery to the skin surface. As expected, the 1.5-mm transducer is more likely to cause this dermal injury. A topical steroid is effective in treating this problem and the authors have not seen any long-term sequelae.[7,12] Although focused ultrasound does not have an affinity for melanin, 2 of 49 Chinese patients treated with Ulthera had transient postinflammatory hyperpigmentation of the forehead in an initial safety study.[24] It has been reported that sensory innervation to the treated areas is also effected in up to 18% of patients.[7] This temporary numbness usually resolves without intervention in 2 to 3 weeks but is variable and can be more pronounced after multiple treatments. As described previously in the authors' personal experience, facial motor nerve injury is possible (**Fig. 9**).[25] Fortunately, full function of the authors' patients' near-total frontal branch paresis returned by 6 months with observation alone. Although rare, other users have reported similar motor nerve complications.

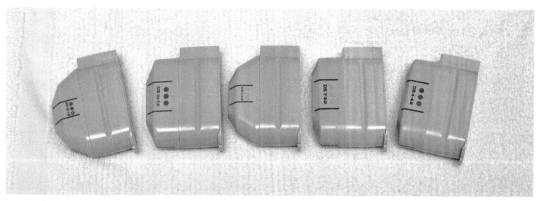

Fig. 7. Ulthera transducers (*left to right*): 10-MHz 1.5-mm narrow, 10-MHz 1.5-mm, 7.0-MHz 3.0 mm-narrow, 7.0-MHz 3.0-mm, and 4.0-MHz 4.5-mm (7.0-MHz 4.5-mm [*not shown*]). (*Courtesy of* Ulthera, Mesa, AZ; with permission.)

POSTPROCEDURE CARE/RECOVERY

Ulthera is a true no-downtime procedure. The authors typically apply a light moisturizer and sunscreen after removal of the ultrasound gel. No specific aftercare is required after this procedure and patients can return to their usual routine right away. Immediately after the treatment, the skin feels tighter to patients. This initial response may shift to visible changes in 3 to 6 months.

OUTCOMES

The authors' experience is based on treating approximately 200 patients to date over the past 3 years in a cosmetic plastic surgery practice. Treatments are almost exclusively performed by aestheticians, including one who is a previous clinical applications specialist for Ulthera. Through critical analysis of the authors' patients' standardized before-and-after treatment images, a variable set of responders and few numbers of patients with aesthetically good results in the neck were found. A good result was defined as improved contour and no evidence of increased skin redundancy after treatment. Patients who achieved a good result approximated the ideal candidate, as described previously. Post-treatment submental lipoptosis reduction was the most consistent finding in these patients (**Fig. 10**). Alternatively, responders with poor elasticity and submental fat reduction led to a poor aesthetic result with increased neck skin and laxity (**Figs. 11** and **12**). This occurred in both ideal and intermediate

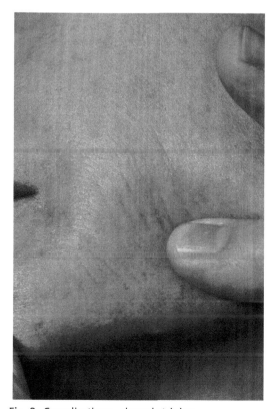

Fig. 8. Complications—dermal striping.

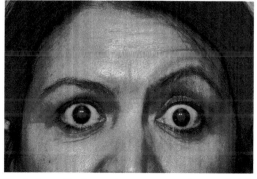

Fig. 9. Complications—temporary weakness of right frontal branch of the facial nerve after off-label treatment of right brow with a 4-MHz 4.5-mm transducer.

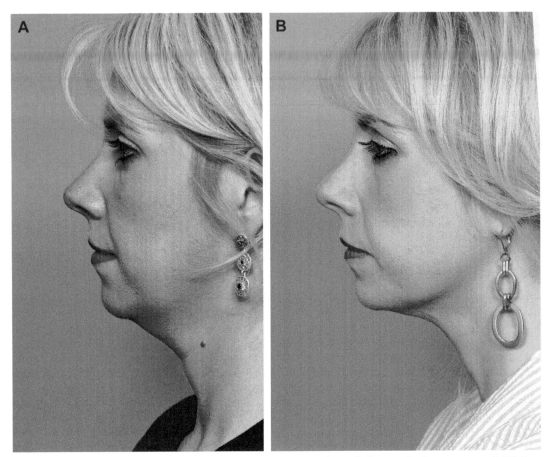

Fig. 10. A 37-year-old woman with submental treatment 13-month result from a single treatment of 180 lines. Lateral images: (*A*) pre and (*B*) 13 month result.

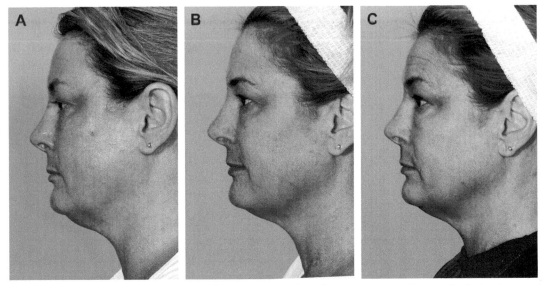

Fig. 11. A 50-year-old woman with lower face/neck 6-month and 1.5-year results from a single treatment of 500 lines. Lateral images: (*A*) pre; (*B*) 6 months; and (*C*) 1.5 year result.

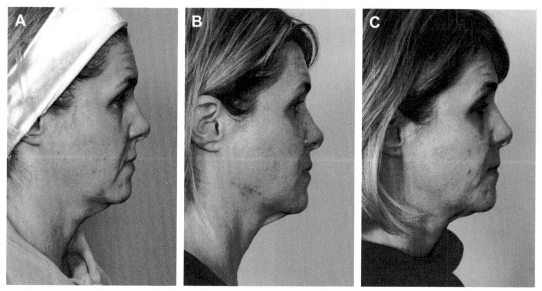

Fig. 12. A 46-year-old woman with lower face/neck 2-year result from a single treatment of 518 lines. Lateral images: (A) pre; (B) 1 year; and (C) 2 year result.

candidates. Overall, in intermediate candidates, consistencies in responses were the most variable (Fig. 13). In this population, the added transducer options, increased line density protocols, and repeat treatments did not predictably improve treatment results or consistency. Similarly, poor candidates rarely had a response, and increased treatment density protocols did not demonstrate a marked difference in results (Figs. 14–16). Contrary to the study by Sasaki and Teves,[21] the

authors' results peaked near 3 months and did not continue to improve at 6 months. In responders, results seemed to wane between 18 months and 2 years in long-term follow-up (Fig. 17).

CLINICAL RESULTS IN THE LITERATURE

As a company, Ulthera seems focused on identifying further treatment applications and improving

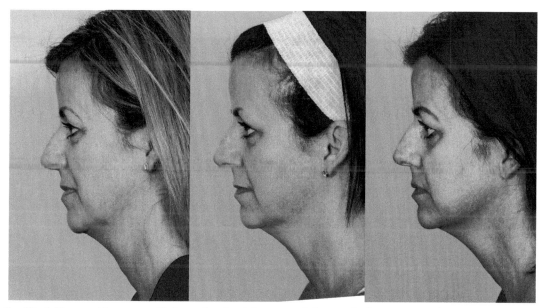

Fig. 13. A 48-year-old woman with lower face/neck 2-year result from a single treatment of 658 lines. Lateral images: (Left to Right) pre, 6-month, and 1-year results.

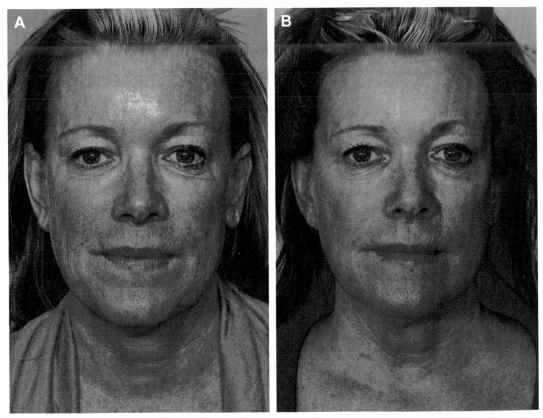

Fig. 14. A 56-year-old woman with lower face/neck 1-year result from a single treatment of 955 lines. Lateral images: (*A*) pre and (*B*) 1 year result.

treatment for comfort and safety. The safety and efficacy of the device in creating focal TCPs within the dermis, subdermis, and SMAS layers without epidermal injury was verified through early porcine and human pilot studies.[9–12] Currently, 36 trials for face and body applications using the device are registered on the National Institutes of Health domain.[26] The results of these studies should help improve the treatments and further support an enthusiastic community of device owners. That said, published literature for peer review on treatment of the neck is limited at this time.

Evidence of clinical utility and approval for a brow lift indication first came from the work of

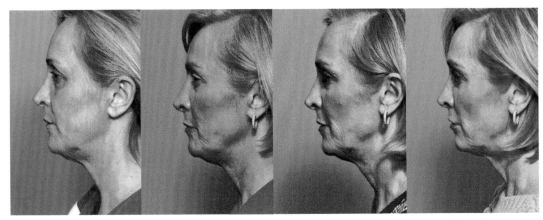

Fig. 15. A 60-year-old woman with lower face/neck 2.5-year result from a single treatment of 415 lines. Lateral images: (*Left to Right*) pre, 1-year, 1.5-year, and 2-year results.

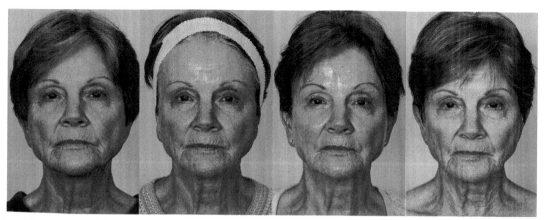

Fig. 16. A 74-year-old woman with lower face/neck 1-year result from a single treatment of 397 lines. Frontal images: (*Left to Right*) pre, 6-month, 1-year, and 1.5-year results.

Alam and colleagues.[13] This prospective cohort study was also the first study to evaluate treatment of the lower face. Unfortunately, the difficulties in finding reliable landmarks for measurements made obtaining data in the lower face difficult. Therefore, results and conclusions were not possible.

Subsequently, Suh and colleagues[7] assessed jawline improvement through Ulthera treatment in a Korean patient population. Lower face treatment consisted of 70 lines to bilateral cheeks and 90 lines to the submentum using the 4.4-MHz 4.5-mm transducer at 1.0 J and the 7.5-MHz 3-mm transducer at 0.45 J. Pre- and post-treatment photograph assessments by 2 reviewers found improvement in each of the 22 patients; 73% of patients reported improvement in their jawline after treatment. A secondary endpoint of histologic change was evaluated by punch biopsy of the treated facial tissue of consenting subjects. Histologic results were assessed for a change in the fraction of collagen and dermal thickness. Findings consisted of patients having 23.7% more dermal collagen fibers

and an increased overall dermal thickness. Also, elastic fibers within the upper and lower reticular dermis were more parallel and straighter.

With a 2-pass protocol in a Korean population, a combination of the 4-MHz 4.5-mm transducer at 1.2 J and the 7-MHz 3.0-mm transducer at 0.63 J were used for treatment of the face and upper neck. An average of 238 lines was delivered. Improvement was evaluated at 90 days in 10 patients. Outcomes were determined by a review of pre- and post-treatment photographs by 2 blinded physicians and patient self-assessments. Clinical improvement was seen in 8 of 10 patients (2 mild, 4 moderate, and 2 significant) by photo review and 9 of 10 (2 mild, 5 moderate, and 2 significant) by patient self-reports.[23] As was seen in the previous study, the subjective physician and patient reports of improvement were better than 80%, but the measurable benefits of a multipass treatments are difficult to determine.

In a safety and efficacy study by Sasaki and Teves,[21] an attempt was made to optimize treatments with regards to treatment vector, energy delivered, and efficacy of multipass protocols.

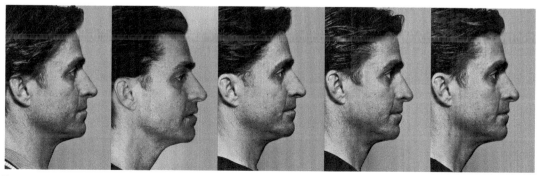

Fig. 17. A 46-year-old man with lower face/neck 1-year result from a single treatment of 830 lines. Lateral images: (*Left to Right*) pre, 3-month, 6-month, and 1-year results.

After 2 pilot studies to determine ideal settings and vectors, a comparison of low- and high-density treatment protocols were compared in 154 patients. Twice the number of lines was used in the high-density group. Although a full face treatment was performed, 75 lines were delivered with both the 7-MHz 3.0-mm and 4-MHz 4.5-mm transducers in the low-density groups. At 6 months, 70.3% of the low-density group and 80.2% of the high-density group were found to be responders by subjective blinded global assessment of the facial aesthetic.[21]

Most recently, Kenkel[15] focused specifically on treatment of the neck, which ultimately led to FDA approval for this indication. In their 70-patient cohort study, a low-density, dual-depth treatment was performed. They used either the 4-MHz 4.5-mm or the 7-MHz 4.5-mm transducer at the deep level and the 7-MHz 3.0-mm transducer at the superficial level. The primary outcome measure was the quantitative change in the submental tissue determined through comparison of standardized pre- and 90-day post-treatment profile images. A response was defined as greater than 20 mm^2 of change in the calculated submental area. With this definition, 72.9% of patients had a response, and the mean change of this subset was approximately 71 mm^2. These findings were supported by masked assessment by 3 clinicians finding improvement in 68.6% of subjects in the submental area and neck at the same endpoint. As a secondary outcome measure, a patient satisfaction questionnaire indicated 67% thought they had improvement.[16,22]

To assess treatment response to increased line density, a more recent study focused on comparison of density and treatment areas for improvement in the neck.[16,22] Three, unequal, nonrandomized groups totaling 64 patients were treated by 1 of 3 protocols: (1) group A—submental dual-depth and lower neck single depth; (2) group B—jowls, submental, and lower neck dual depth; (3) group C—submental and lower neck dual depth. A qualitative photo comparison by 3 reviewers at 90 days post-treatment resulted in group A having the most patients with improvement at 53% and groups B and C with 41% (after data removal for poor photos, adjusted results of 63% group A and 46% groups B and C). As a secondary measure, patient self-evaluations and physician clinical evaluations were used to complete a 5-point subjective global aesthetic improvement scale (GAIS) at 60, 90, and 180 days. The subject and physician GAIS ranged from 40% to 96% improvement, but the results were highly variable and made drawing conclusions difficult. Finally, a patient satisfaction questionnaire was used, in which higher overall satisfaction was noted in group C at both 90 and 180 days post-treatment than in groups A or B. In the authors' opinion, the conclusion that dual-depth treatment is objectively better than single-depth treatment is not supported from the results, irrespective of higher patient satisfaction.

DISCUSSION

With a straightforward design and changes in the software, Ulthera is easy to use and amenable to treatments by staff with supervision in a medical spa setting. The growing desire for a no-downtime treatment option for face (and possibly the body) may expand the utility of the device and candidates for the procedure. Additionally, return on investment is high with cost of consumables ($0.88/line) far lower than typical fees charged for treatments rendered. Time required by staff for treatments can also be factored into the total cost in addition to a per-line model or as an alternative to flat rate pricing. Therefore, the device is financially appealing in a medical practice with a cosmetic focus, both with or without surgical treatment options.

As practitioners, the authors' early enthusiasm has waned from lack of substantial, predictable results in practice. Through early studies, it is clear the Ulthera device does safely and effectively deliver focused tissue disruption at multiple tissue depths, sparing the dermis. Translation of tissue injury to a clinical improvement in the neck is not as transparent. Despite some good early responses using low treatment densities in a few ideal candidates, the authors have quickly adopted increased line density and multilevel treatment protocols in an attempt to obtain reproducible, aesthetically pleasing, visible results. From a theoretic standpoint, more lines and energy delivered should lead to an increase in the wound healing response, more collagen deposition, improved elastosis, and more lipolysis, leading to better contours. In the authors' experience, increased line density has not increased the percentage of responders or overcome the limitations presented by patient anatomy. In those patients who are responders, it is unclear if more energy delivered is directly related to a more substantial result than would have been achieved at lower densities. An objective study of the neck with measurable outcomes has yet to be published in the literature to support these increased density protocols. High-density protocols also add substantial cost to patients because time and disposable costs multiply with double- and triple-level treatments, requiring approximately 530 or 790 lines, respectively. Full face treatments including the neck may require more than 1000 lines.

In the published studies to date, even with careful patient selection (good health, mild to moderate rhytids/laxity, normal body mass index, lack of severe elastosis, nonsmoking history, and so forth), variability is a problem.[21,23] This makes recommendations and counseling patients on expected improvement with Ulthera in the lower face somewhat difficult. Mild volume reduction and tightening can be achieved but is variable among patients. The authors are careful in pretreatment counseling to properly manage patient expectations and to educate patients that their healing response largely determines their results. In patients who are deemed intermediate, the limitations in their anatomic findings or history are further explained. Poor candidates are routinely dissuaded from the procedure and rarely treated.

From an objective standpoint, comparing the results from the authors' surgical methods to those obtained with the Ulthera device, there is frequently a disappointment. Therefore, giving recommendations on the best treatment option becomes difficult when patients truly desire and need a surgical result to reach their goals but are hopeful they can achieve it with less expense and no downtime. From a downtime standpoint, only Ulthera and other noninvasive modalities can deliver a true no-downtime option. From a cost perspective, the best option is less clear. In good candidates, submental lipoptosis is the focus of treatment and costs are $2000 to $3000 for a higher-density face treatment, with no guarantee of response and the possibility of a recurrent expense for needed retreatment. Alternatively, submental liposuction affords a single-session treatment with immediate, substantial improvement but is approximately double the cost depending on the region. In the authors' experience, in patients who are poor candidates, a full treatment is one-third to one-quarter the cost of a surgical facelift solution but is unlikely to lead to a clinical response. The authors' beliefs are that the right recommendation is the one that best fits a patient's goals and is straightforward about the limitations of current noninvasive treatments.

The authors continue to offer Ulthera treatments to those patients most likely to achieve a good result and look forward to completion of ongoing studies and publication to support increased treatment density and support the value in these protocols for the neck. A 3-D analysis might offer the offer best methodology for analysis to objectively calculate these small changes difficult to capture with conventional photography. The authors are also looking to better quantify patient satisfaction through questionnaires and have begun looking at combined noninvasive treatment modalities using Ulthera and radiofrequency to achieve more reliable results. Ultimately, the goal continues to provide the best outcomes and value to patients even with nonsurgical treatment offerings. Although it fills a niche in the authors' practice, the authors continue to evaluate this technology to confirm that it adds to patient satisfaction and willingness to consider the authors' services for their family, friends, business colleagues, and acquaintances for their plastic surgical needs.

SUPPLEMENTARY DATA

Supplementary data related to this article can be found online at http://dx.doi.org/10.1016/j.fsc.2014.01.011.

REFERENCES

1. Hayashi K, Thabit G III, Massa KL, et al. The effect of thermal heating on the length and histological properties of the glenohumeral joint capsule. Am J Sports Med 1997;25:107–12.

2. Fry WJ, Wulff VJ, Tucker D, et al. Physical factors in ultrasonically induced changes in living systems: I. Identification of non-temperature effects. J Acoust Soc Am 1950;22:867–76.

3. Fry WJ. Intense ultrasound: a new tool for neurological research. J Ment Sci 1954;22:85–96.

4. Jolesz FA. MRI-guided focused ultrasound surgery. Annu Rev Med 2009;60:417–30.

5. Jolesz FA, Hynynen K, McDannold N, et al. MR imaging–Controlled focused ultrasound ablation: a noninvasive image-guided surgery. Magn Reson Imaging Clin N Am 2005;13:545–60.

6. Clement GT. Perspectives in clinical uses of high-intensity focused ultrasound. Ultrasonics 2004;42:1087–93.

7. Suh DH, Shin MK, Lee JS, et al. Intense focused ultrasound tightening in asian skin: clinical and pathologic results. Dermatol Surg 2011;37:1595–602.

8. U.S. Food and Drug Administration, Center for Drug Evaluation and Research. ExAblate 2000 System P040003 approval letter. 2004. Available at: http://www.accessdata.fda.gov/cdrh_docs/pdf4/P040003a.pdf. Accessed November 1, 2011.

9. White WM, Makin IR, Slayton MH, et al. Selective transcutaneous delivery of energy to porcine soft tissues using intense ultrasound. Lasers Surg Med 2008;40:67–75.

10. White WM, Makin IR, Barthe PG, et al. Selective creation of thermal injury zones in the superficial musculoaponeurotic system using intense ultrasound therapy: a new target for noninvasive facial rejuvenation. Arch Facial Plast Surg 2007;9:22–9.

11. Laubach HJ, Makin IR, Barthe PG, et al. Intense focused ultrasound: evaluation of a new treatment modality for precise microcoagulation within the skin. Dermatol Surg 2008;34.727–34.

12. Gliklich RE, White WM, Slayton MH, et al. Clinical pilot study of intense ultrasound therapy to deep dermal facial skin and subcutaneous tissues. Arch Facial Plast Surg 2007;9:88–95.

13. Alam M, White LE, Martin NE, et al. Ultrasound tightening of facial and neck skin: a rater-blinded prospective cohort study. J Am Acad Dermatol 2010; 62:262–9.

14. U.S. Food and Drug Administration, Center for Drug Evaluation and Research. Ulthera K072505 approval letter. 2009. Available at: www.accessdata.fda.gov/cdrh_docs/pdf7/K072505.pdf. Accessed November 1, 2011.

15. Kenkel J. Evaluation of the Ulthera system for improving skin laxity and tightening. Abstract presentation, ASAPS Annual Meeting. Vancouver (Canada), May 3–8, 2012.

16. Lower Face Submentum and Neck. Ultherapy white paper. 2013. Available at: http://www.ultherapy.com/uploads/document/public/Lower_Face_Submentum_and_Neck_1001890C.pdf. Accessed November 20, 2013.

17. U.S. Food and Drug Administration, Center for Drug Evaluation and Research. Ulthera K121700 approval letter. 2012. Available at: www.accessdata.fda.gov/cdrh_docs/pdf12/K121700.pdf. Accessed August 3, 2012.

18. Sunderam H. Propective double-blind, randomized pilot study comparing ibuprofen to a narcotic for pain management during micro-focused ultrasound treatment. Oral presentation, ASDS Annual Meeting. 2011, Washington, DC, November 4, 2011.

19. Gitt S. Double-blind, randomized, controlled split-face trial to assess the efficacy and safety of a liposomal lidocaine topical for pain management during micro-focused ultrasound treatment. Poster Presentation, Aesthetic Meeting. Vancouver (Canada), May 4, 2012.

20. Ulthera. 2012. Comfort Management [White Paper] Mesa, AZ: Print 1001182Doc Rev. A.

21. Sasaki GH, Teves A. Clinical efficacy and safety of focus-imaged ultrasonography: a two year experience. Aesthet Surg J 2012;32:601–12.

22. Ulthera. 2013. Treatment Density [White Paper] Mesa, AZ: Print 1001504Doc Rev. D.

23. Lee HS, Jang WS, Cha YJ, et al. Multiple pass ultrasound tightening of skin laxity of the lower face and neck. Dermatol Surg 2012;38:20–7.

24. Chan NP, Shek SY, Yu CS, et al. Safety study of transcutaneous focused ultrasound for non-invasive skin tightening in Asians. Lasers Surg Med 2011;43:366–75.

25. Brobst RW, Ferguson M, Perkins SW. Ulthera: initial and 6 months results. Facial Plast Surg Clin North Am 2012;20:163–76.

26. U.S. National Institute of Health, Clinical Trials Registry. Available at: http://clinicaltrials.gov/ct2/results?term=ulthera&Search=Search. Accessed November 20, 2013.

Neck Skin Rejuvenation

J. Kevin Duplechain, MD

KEYWORDS

- CO_2 laser • Croton oil peel • Epidermal ablation • Laser resurfacing • Neck lines • Neck lift
- Photodamage • Postoperative wound care

KEY POINTS

- Laser rejuvenation of the neck with the ultrapulsed CO_2 laser provides improvement in tone and texture of treated skin and can be used safely as an adjunct to neck/facelift surgery.
- A novel post-treatment plan with perfluorodecalin emulsion greatly reduces adverse effects traditionally associated with fully ablative resurfacing.
- The croton oil peel technique can be modified (ie, by varying the concentration of croton oil) to affect the depth of penetration, providing unprecedented control of treatment depth and minimizing the likelihood of hypopigmentation.
- The risk of adverse effects during CO_2 laser resurfacing of the neck is reduced by adjusting the treatment parameters to accommodate the reduced healing capacity of the neck compared with the face.

INTRODUCTION

The aging neck is characterized by platysmal bands, lipodystophy, and jowls that extend into the neck.[1] As jowls develop, the chin and jawline lose definition and horizontal and radial necklines become more noticeable.[2] Like the face, the neck is subject to photodamage.[3,4] For these reasons, patients who seek facial rejuvenation often want their neck treated as well to obtain a homogenous, natural appearing improvement in photodamage.[3] Surgical approaches to addressing these and related cervical deformities have been described.[1,5] Nonsurgical modalities, such as botulinum toxins, chemical peels and dermabrasion, radiofrequency energy, plasma skin regeneration (PSR), lasers, and light,[6,7] have also emerged to rejuvenate the skin of both face and neck. Resurfacing of the neck combined with facelift and other surgical procedures must be executed carefully and with significant caution due to the inherent healing limitations of the neck.

BOTULINUM TOXINS

Botulinum toxins have been used to treat vertical platysmal bands[2,8–11] and horizontal neck rhytids.[2,10,11] Results appear within several days and persist for up to 6 months.[6] Potential complications are minimal but include dysphagia and immunoresistance, which may be avoided by using the smallest effective doses, injecting at intervals of at least 3 months, and avoiding booster injections.[8] Careful injection technique is critical to avoid diffusion of toxin to nontargeted muscles near the injection site.[10]

Patients likely to benefit from botulinum toxins should have good cervical skin elasticity, well-defined platysmal bands, and minimal fat descent.[10] The treatment is suitable for older patients who are either poor candidates for surgery or have already had neck rejuvenation surgery. Younger patients with strong platysmal bands that do not require surgery are also candidates.[9] No improvement is expected, however, in the appearance of photodamaged skin.

Disclosure: Dr J.K. Duplechain is a funded speaker for Lumenis Inc, Santa Clara, CA, and a founder and stockholder of Cutagenesis, Lafayette, LA, USA.
1103 Kaliste Saloom Road, Suite 300, Lafayette, LA 70508, USA
E-mail address: jkdmd@drduplechain.com

Facial Plast Surg Clin N Am 22 (2014) 203–216
http://dx.doi.org/10.1016/j.fsc.2014.01.002

PEELS AND DERMABRASION

Although inexpensive, chemical peels and derm-abrasion have produced variable results in photo-damaged facial skin due to the difficulty in controlling the depth of tissue removal.[12] In the neck, dermabrasion and chemical peels are associated with a high risk of scarring,[13] although this risk may be smaller with superficial peels.[6] Roy[6] uses α- and β-hydroxy acid peels to treat vascular and pigmented lesions and fine rhytids on the neck and chest because these peels can be used on all types of skin and there is no down-time. Roy cautions, however, that results are less dramatic than with light and laser treatments. When resurfacing the face with medium to deep peels, Roy uses the Jessner peel on the neck and chest to minimize the transition between the face and neck. Despite side effects and com-plications,[13–15] chemical peeling and dermabra-sion have produced dramatic, long-lasting clinical and histologic improvements in the face.[12,16–19] Superficial peels (eg, α-hydroxy acids) and medium-strength peels, however, have little effect on fine wrinkles.[20] With α- and β-hydroxy peels there is no downtime and these peels can be used on the necks of all skin types.[6] These peels provide no lasting change to skin ultrastructure. When using medium to deep chemical peels to rejuvenate the face, the use of Jessner peel on the neck may minimize the transition from the treated face to the untreated neck.[6] (The neck often remains untreated with medium or deep peels for fear of scarring or hypopigmentation.)

One type of chemical peel has received consid-erable study by Hetter[21–24] and Bensimon.[25] The croton oil peel has been shown to produce consis-tently excellent cosmetic results, even in the neck. This peel evolved from the classic Baker-Gordon peel (phenol and croton oil) reported in 1962[26] and is still used by some physicians. Although the Baker-Gordon peel provided dramatic improvement, its use was sometimes limited because hypopigmentation and a waxy porcelain appearance often resulted after treatment. In 2000, Hetter[21] showed that the active ingredient was croton oil rather than phenol. Hetter further showed that lowering the concentration of phenol, varying the concentration of croton oil, and using a specific application technique permitted surgeons to control the depth of penetration during treat-ment. Thus, surgeons could treat facial areas of different skin thickness, even the eyelids.[25] A com-plete protocol for the modern croton oil peel in facial rejuvenation (including the neck) has been published[25] and is summarized.

CROTON OIL PEEL

Patient selection is critical to the success of croton acid peels. Patients tolerate the peel better if they know what to expect, especially after a procedure is completed. Prospective candidates are shown photographs of patients in various recovery stages and the candidates may also have an opportunity to speak with previous peel patients. With the neck, the goal is to blend skin color with that of the more aggressively treated face rather than to remove wrinkles.[25]

When a patient consents to treatment with a croton oil peel, the neck skin is first treated with tretinoin 1% once daily, beginning 4 to 6 weeks before peeling. If the skin becomes irritated, the frequency is reduced. Hydroquinone 4% is applied twice daily to prevent postinflammatory hyperpig-mentation, and glycolic acid 8% is given once daily to facilitate exfoliation. These preparatory treatments are stopped 4 to 5 days before peeling. By that time, the skin is erythematous and flaky and patients have been told this is normal. Antiviral medication is routinely started 3 days before peeling and continued for 1 week after peeling to prevent herpetic complications.[25]

For the thin skin of the neck, a croton oil 0.1% solution is prepared by dilution of the croton oil 0.2% solution, which is, in turn, prepared from a stock solution of phenol (35% by volume) and croton oil (4%) as described.[25] The 0.1% croton oil peel is a light peel and affects only the epidermis. The peel solution is applied by sequen-tial light applications with gauze and cotton-tipped applicators. The acid precipitates skin protein to form a white frost in 10 to 20 seconds. The depth of penetration is judged by the degree of frosting. As discussed previously, the concentration of croton oil and the application technique are the primary determinants of penetration depth. The endpoint of treatment is the degree of frosting, which is a subjective and experience-based judg-ment. Outcomes are optimized when practitioners have sufficient experience to recognize when the appropriate depth is reached as revealed by the frost. For the neck, the light peel results in a "light, wispy frost that is not at all organized."[25]

When the frosting subsides, an emulsion of Pol-ysporin (Pfizer, New York, New York) and lidocaine jelly is applied over the peeled areas and given to patients for continued use. The mixture moistur-izes the peeled area, prevents crusting, and pro-vides analgesia. Postpeel medication includes a narcotic agent for pain, ibuprofen, Medrol Dose-pak (Mova Pharmaceutical, Manati, Puerto Rico), and, if necessary, a sleep medication. Healing is complete in 2 weeks, although erythema persists for up to 12 weeks. If healing is delayed and the peeled areas thicken with mild scarring, peeling probably penetrated to the deep reticular dermis. In this event, triamcinolone acetonide and 5-fluorouracil are injected. Hyperpigmentation, if it occurs during recovery, is temporary and treated with tretinoin and hydroquinone 4%.[25]

In summary, the croton oil peel is an inexpensive and effective modality for rejuvenating neck skin because the technique can be modified (ie, by varying the concentration of croton oil) to affect the depth of penetration, thus providing surgeons with unprecedented control of treatment depth and minimizing the likelihood of hypopigmentation.[25] Bensimon's current use of the croton oil peel is limited to the upper cervical skin just above the first cervical crease to prevent a noticeable transition from face to neck (Richard Bensimon, MD, personal communication, June 2013).

PLASMA SKIN REGENERATION

PSR has been shown to improve moderately photodamaged skin of the face,[27] neck, chest, and hands.[7] Plasma is an ionized gas produced when electrons are removed from atoms. The PSR device includes an ultra–high-frequency radiofrequency generator that imparts energy to inert nitrogen gas in a hand piece. Energy is delivered to the target tissue at different depths without dependence on skin chromophores. Treatment requires the use of topical anesthesia, oral anesthesia, or both, depending on the amount of energy. Alster and Konda[7] obtained mean clinical improvements of 41%, 48%, and 57% in the neck, hands, and chest, respectively, up to 3 months after a single treatment. Wrinkle severity and hyperpigmentation were significantly reduced and skin smoothness was significantly improved in all 3 areas. Side effects were limited to edema, erythema, and desquamation. To the author's knowledge, the PSR device, although used by some physicians, is no longer commercially available.

LASERS

A variety of laser and light-based procedures have been used to rejuvenate neck skin (**Table 1**). Considered the gold standard for rejuvenating skin, the ablative CO_2 laser ushered in an era of precision and thus the possibility of better predictability compared with chemical peels and dermabrasion. As discussed later, early attempts at neck resurfacing were marred by complications due to treatment and technologic issues. With multigenerational improvements and better understanding of treatment nuances, however, successful treatments are now consistently achievable. The CO_2 laser emits light at 10,600-nm and targets tissue water, which absorbs energy at this wavelength. A single pulse ablates the upper 20 μm of skin and collateral damage occurs at 0.2- to 1.0-mm depths.[28,29] Advantages include control of tissue vaporization, minimal excessive residual thermal damage, dermal collagen contraction, and hemostasis.[12]

The CO_2 laser for neck skin rejuvenation has been studied by 4 groups.[30–33] All used 1 or 2 passes with anesthesia and 100- to 500-mJ energy. Moderate improvements were noted in skin color, texture, tightening, and rhytids whereas adverse effects were transient and limited to erythema, hyperpigmentation, hypopigmentation, and, in the lower neck, scarring. In their 308-patient study, Behroozan and colleagues[31] showed that a short-pulsed CO_2 laser could safely rejuvenate the neck and the face at the same time with minimal risk of scarring or permanent pigmentary changes. Fitzpatrick and colleagues[32] pointed out that wound healing of the neck, especially in the lower third, is noticeably less satisfactory than healing of the face. Healing is also more satisfactory in the upper neck than in the lower neck, so the lower part of the neck may require different treatment settings, as suggested earlier by Rosenberg.[34] Consistent with these findings, Sasaki and colleagues[35] reported average skin depths of 115 μm, 75 μm, and 70 μm for the upper, mid, and lower neck, respectively, and corresponding adnexal densities, all of which suggest that laser treatment settings for upper neck differ significantly from the treatment parameters used for the mid and lower neck.

The rationale for using the 2940-nm Er:YAG laser to resurface the neck is based on an anticipated reduction in thermal damage[3,20,36] compared with the CO_2 laser. Because 2940 nm is at the peak of water absorption, diffusion of heat to surrounding tissue is greatly reduced, thus lowering the risk of scarring and damage to pilosebaceous units. As shown in **Table 1**, energies were higher (600–1700 mJ) than with the CO_2 laser and 1 to 4 passes were made. Improvements were variable (0%–75%) and adverse effects included temporary erythema and hyperpigmentation. In 1 case,[3] erythema was secondary to infection. Although use of anesthesia was not reported by 2 groups,[3,20] patients of Jimenez and Spencer[4] required topical anesthesia before treatment and local infiltration of lidocaine during Er:YAG laser resurfacing of the neck.

Goldman and Marchell[36] treated the necks of 11 patients with a near-simultaneous beam of

Table 1
Rejuvenation of neck skin with laser and light-based therapies

Reference (No. Patients)	Treatment Parameters	Results	Adverse Effects	Comments
CO₂ Laser				
Fanous et al,[30] 1998 (n = 48)	100–175 mJ, 1 pass; 35% overlap for upper, 20% for lower and lateral areas; treatment parameters lower than on face	Improved rhytids, skin color, tightness, but less than face; skin color and texture similar to face; high patient satisfaction	Transient erythema, hyperpigmentation, hypopigmentation	Topical/block local anesthesia; average follow-up 11 mo
Behroozan et al,[31] 2000 (n = 308)	90-μs Pulse duration, 500 mJ, 3-mm spot size, 2 passes (entire neck, no scanner)	39% Improvement in rhytids and tightening, 85% of patients pleased	Transient hyperpigmentation, erythema	Local IV sedation or general anesthesia, 6–18 mo follow-up, absence of complications attributed to short pulse duration
Fitzpatrick et al,[32] 2001 (n = 10)	1 Pass with laser equipped with CPG, 300 mJ with CPG at pattern 3, size 9, density 6	Moderate improvement in color and texture, no improvement in wrinkling	Mild hypopigmented scarring in lower neck, erythema	Anterior and anterolateral skin treated, deep intravenous sedation, 3–6 mo follow-up
Kilmer et al,[33] 2003 (n = 100)	300 mJ, 60 W, energy density 1–3, 1 pass	Rhytids, texture, pigmentary changes improved, blending of skin color when face and neck treated together	Erythema, whitening, postinflammatory hyperpigmentation, hypopigmentation (rare)	Preoperative lidocaine/prilocaine hydration necessary; epidermis not wiped after treatment, avoided overlapping or stacking pulses
Er:YAG Laser				
Goldberg & Meine,[20] 1998 (n = 10)	300-μs Pulse duration, 5-mm spot size, 600–800 mJ, 3000–4500 mJ/cm², 5–10 Hz, 10% overlap, 4 passes to mild bleeding	25% Improvement in rhytids, 50% improvement in pigmentary stigmata	Transient erythema	Anesthesia not used, follow-up limited to 6 mo, healing complete in 10 d, no wiping of debris between passes
Goldman et al,[3] 1999 (n = 20)	Method 1: 5-mm collimated beam, 8700 mJ/cm² (1 pass) followed by 0.2-mm noncollimated spot and 1700 mJ (defocused mode), spot size 5–10 mm, fluence 2000–9000 mJ/cm², 1 pass Method 2: 4-mm noncollimated spot, 1700 mJ (13,5000 mJ/cm²), 1 pass to entire neck followed by second pass at same settings to upper half of neck; more defocused pass (6–10 mm spot size, 2000–6000 mJ/cm²) to lower half of neck	Method 1: skin texture and skin color 28% improvement Method 2: skin texture 48% improvement, skin color 45% improvement	Persistent erythema secondary to infection (n = 1)	Healing complete in 7–10 d, 3 mo follow-up, anesthesia use not reported

Study	Parameters	Results	Complications	Notes
Jimenez & Spencer,[4] 1999 (n = 5)	1000 mJ (500 mJ/cm²), 5-mm Spot size, 1-2 passes	Improvement variable: 0%-25% (n = 3), 25%-50% (n = 1), 50%-75% (n = 1)	Transitory hyperpigmentation	2-3 wk to heal, topical anesthesia and local infiltration of lidocaine, 6-mo follow-up
CO₂/Er:YAG Laser Combination				
Goldman & Marchell et al,[36] 1999 (n = 11)	Er:YAG: 4-mm spot, 16,000 mJ/cm²; CO₂: 5 W, 50-ms pulse, 2 passes	Skin color, moderate improvement, skin texture and wrinkling, greater improvement, patient satisfaction higher with CO₂-Er:YAG than with Er:YAG alone	None observed	3-6 mo follow-up, anesthesia not reported, debris not removed between passes
Intense Pulsed Light				
Weiss et al,[37] 2002 (n = 80)	Broadband light, 570-nm cutoff filter, double pulses (2.4 ms, 10-ms delay, 6 ms), 30,000-40,000 J/cm²; cool gel during treatment	71% of patients with improved skin texture, reduced telangiectasia, or more uniform pigmentation	Long-lasting hypopigmentation (2.5%), temporary mild crusting, erythema, purpura	4-Year follow-up after several treatments
Nonablative 1540-nm Er:Glass Laser				
Dahan et al,[38] 2004 (n = 20)	10,000 mJ/cm² per pulse, 3 pulses. 2-hz repetition rate, 4-mm spot hand piece. contact cooling, 5 treatments	Improved skin tone and texture, dermal thickness increased by 110 µm (due to increase in collagen fibers), all patients extremely satisfied	None observed	3-Month follow-up after 5th treatment
Ablative Fractional CO₂ Laser				
Tierney et al,[55] 2011 (n = 10)	20 W, 500 pitch, 500 ms, contact cooling; 1-3 treatments at 6- to 8-week interval	Skin texture 62.9% improvement, skin laxity 57.0%, rhytids 51.4%, overall cosmetic outcome 59.3%	Temporary edema, erythema, pruritis	2-Month follow-up

Abbreviation: CPG, computerized pattern generator.
Data from Refs.[3,4,20,30-33,36-39]

low-fluence CO_2 and Er:YAG laser energies. The investigators had previously observed that nonspecific thermal damage with the combination beam was 14.8 to 37 μm, which is less than that of the CO_2 laser alone (27.2–59.2 μm) or the Er:YAG immediately after CO_2 resurfacing (22.6–37 μm). They found that improvement in skin texture and color was greater with the combined beam than with the Er:YAG alone. Patient satisfaction was also higher and adverse events were not observed, suggesting that the CO_2/Er:YAG laser beam was more suitable for neck resurfacing than the Er:YAG laser alone.

Weiss and colleagues[37] reported a 4-year study of patients treated several times with intense pulsed light. Improvement was noted in skin texture, telangiectasia, and pigmentation while adverse effects included transient crusting, erythema, and purpura. Long-lasting hypopigmentation was noted in 2.5% of patients. Dahan and colleagues,[38] using a nonablative Er:Glass laser, obtained improvement in skin texture and tone and increased dermal thickness, which they attributed to the growth of collagen fibers. Patients received 5 treatments. Adverse effects were not observed.

Using an ablative fractional CO_2 laser, Tierney and Hanke[39] obtained improvement in overall cosmesis as well as skin texture, laxity, and rhytids with minimal adverse effects. In fractional technology, the laser beam creates an array of microscopic wounds at specific depths rather than vaporizing the entire outer layer of tissue. Collateral damage is controlled and healing is rapid because the tissue surrounding each tiny wound is undamaged and keratinocytes have only short distances to migrate during re-epithelialization. Collagen contracts and neocollagenesis are initiated.[40,41]

The advantages of fractional over fully ablative lasers are documented. Re-epithelialization after treatment is more rapid, post-treatment skin care is shorter, acneiform eruptions are less frequent, and postoperative erythema resolves more quickly.[39,42] Adverse effects of fractional ablative lasers have only recently been reported. Avram and coworkers,[42] for example, described hypertrophic scarring of the neck in 5 patients who had recently undergone fractional laser treatment. The investigators suggested that the scars might be attributed to the neck's low wound-healing capacity, a "subtle fibrosis" due to damaged blood vessels after face or neck lift surgery, or a plastic surgery procedure in which underprivileged neck skin was placed on the face. Shamsaldeen and colleagues[43] reported adverse events in 16.8% of 374 patients treated on the neck, face, and

other nonfacial areas with a deep fractional CO_2 laser. Adverse effects have also been found on the neck and other areas treated with the 1500-nm erbium-doped fractional laser.[10]

A CASE OF COMPLICATIONS IN FRACTIONAL LASER RESURFACING

A case in which adverse effects were observed after fractional CO_2 laser resurfacing provided elsewhere is described. The author also provides a plausible explanation for these complications and recommends treatment modifications to minimize the risk of their occurrence.

Case

A 45-year-old woman presented with tightness, inflammation, and erythema in neck skin that had worsened 4 days after treatment with a fractional CO_2 laser (Solta Medical, Inc [formerly Reliant Technologies], Hayward, California). The patient had previously undergone 2 facial fractional resurfacing procedures without incident. Treatment parameters of the neck laser procedure were 40 mJ and 36% density under topical anesthesia. Initial consultation was obtained via telephone 4 days after the resurfacing treatment because the patient had undergone treatment in another state. Silver sulfadiazine (Silvadene) was the initial treatment prescribed by local emergency department professionals at the author's recommendation. The patient was started on a topical perfluorodecalin emulsion (Cutagenix, Cutagenesis, Lafayette, Louisiana) 4 times daily and 2 days later Silvadene was discontinued. The patient has continued to improve for more than 1 year but still demonstrates moderate scarring. The patient is shown in **Fig. 1.**

Discussion

This case shows that when neck and facial skin are treated aggressively with a fractional CO_2 laser, significant complications may occur. These treatment parameters correlate with depth of penetration into the reticular dermis at approximately 800 μm. These findings corroborate those of earlier reports[42,44] in which treatment parameters ranged from 15 to 70 mJ and 20% to 45% density. Avram and colleagues[42] attributed their adverse effects to the excessive treatment conditions. They suggested that scarring in their study may have been due to thermal injury resulting from overlap of high-energy CO_2 application. Fife and coworkers[44] also suggested that their adverse effects were attributable to high energy, density, or both.

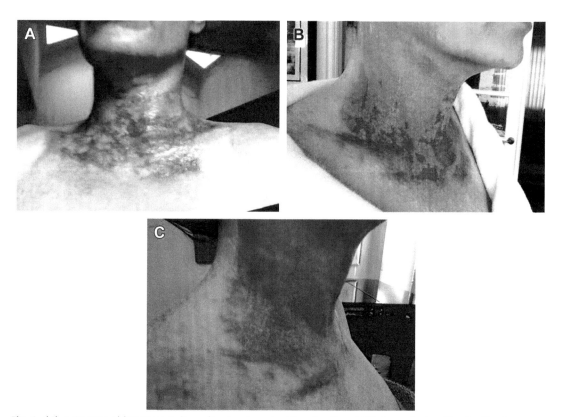

Fig. 1. (*A*) A 44-year-old woman 4 days after treatment with a fractional CO_2 laser device. The depth of penetration was 900 μm and the treatment density was 35%. Note the significant degree of second- and third-degree burns within the treatment area. Despite the fractional nature of this treatment, significant injury occurred beyond that expected at 35% treatment density, resulting in an expanded density approaching 100% of the treated area. (*B*) The same patient on day 8, 1 day after starting perfluorodecalin emulsion and (*C*) 6 days after start of the emulsion.

The consequences of overlap, or spread of energy during fractional laser resurfacing, may be understood by considering pulse duration, which plays an important role in collateral thermal damage during ablative CO_2 laser resurfacing and was well described in the study of lasered pig skin.[45] Pulses longer than 1 millisecond are known to increase thermal damage.[46] The concept is illustrated in **Fig. 2**.

The energy necessary to ablate biologic tissue (ie, the ablation threshold), however, is fixed for a given type of tissue. In fractional laser resurfacing, pulse durations equal to or less than 0.8 millisecond result in a narrow zone of thermal damage.[47] As pulse duration increases, the ablative and thermal zones become wider, causing the diameter of each zone to increase. Consequently, the thermal zones may become continuous, and the treatment could become fully ablative.

In the case described previously, the fractional treatment injured the reticular dermis, a tissue layer known to have fewer skin adnexa (particularly in

the neck) to aid in healing. To reach the depth of the reticular dermis, the pulse duration had to have been increased, resulting in wider thermal zones and greater zones of ablation, thus increasing the actual density of treatment. These factors could have contributed to the unexpected complications in the patient. In an unpublished case of another patient (**Fig. 3**) treated by the author, high pulse frequency during fractional CO_2 laser resurfacing is believed to have caused increased dermal heating, resulting in prolonged erythema and scarring. This explanation is reasonable, because varied pulse frequency rates have been observed to correspond with increased or prolonged erythema in superpulsed CO_2 laser treatments.[48]

The author agrees with the suggestion of Avram and coworkers[42] that scarring in their study may have been due to thermal injury resulting from overlap and deep reticular dermal injury of a high-energy CO_2 application, because such energy would result in double-treating and

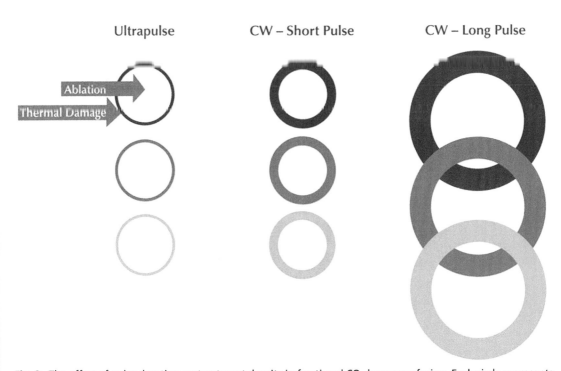

Fig. 2. The effect of pulse duration on treatment density in fractional CO_2 laser resurfacing. Each circle represents a microthermal wound created by the fractional laser beam. The pulse duration is shortest with the high-energy CO_2 laser and longest with the low-energy continuous wave (CW) laser. The circumferential lines represent the areas of thermal damage (ie, thick lines denote greater thermal damage than thin lines). As the desired depth of penetration is increases, zones of thermal injury also increase as a result of the prolonged pulse width necessary to achieve the desired depth. This phenomenon becomes more clinically relevant when pulse width exceeds the TRT of skin (0.8–1.0 ms). In the most extreme case, fractional treatments may become fully ablative due to the overlap in thermal zones, as shown in the diagram on the far right. This effect is believed to account for the unexpected adverse effects at long pulse durations of fractional resurfacing procedures.

subsequent adverse effects. The author, therefore, recommends that treatment densities in fractional CO_2 laser resurfacing be limited to 15% (per pass) to reduce the risk of complications, especially in areas with few adnexal structures, such as the neck. Additional recommendations include limiting depth of penetration with small spot size (120 μm) fractional devices to the papillary or upper reticular dermis and considering the use of a larger spot size (1.3 mm) for fractional resurfacing in epidermal ablation. Finally, frequency should be considered as a variable known to increase erythema and prolong healing when excessive. These precautions have proved valuable in minimizing unexpected complications in the author's practice.

NECK REJUVENATION WITH THE ABLATIVE CO_2 LASER

Despite the growth of nonablative devices, the author uses an ultrapulsed CO_2 laser (UltraPulse CO_2, Lumenis, San Jose, California) to rejuvenate facial and neck skin. The adverse effects of ablative CO_2 lasers—prolonged erythema, pruritis, hyperpigmentation and hypopigmentation, acne flares, milia, contact dermatitis, infections, pain during treatment, and scarring—are well documented.[12,30,49–53] These reports of complications related to ablative resurfacing, although still real, represent treatment series with first- or second-generation devices. Newer devices with shorter pulse width and treatment parameters better designed for specific anatomic areas make ablative resurfacing on and off the face a more favorable treatment option than perhaps once considered. Treatment parameters must be modified to account for the differences in the skin structure throughout the face and neck. For example, the risk of scarring is greater in the neck than in the face because the neck has fewer pilosebaceous units than the face, and the epidermis and dermis are both thinner.[54] By treating these anatomic areas uniquely, the author has been able to

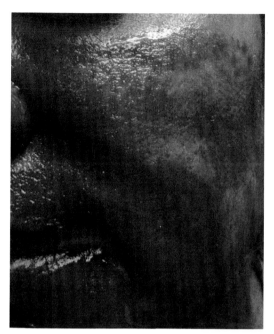

Fig. 3. A patient previously treated elsewhere by fractional CO_2 laser resurfacing at high pulse frequency, resulting in increased dermal heating, prolonged erythema, and scarring in the treated area.

successfully develop protocols, which allow CO_2 resurfacing of the neck with minimal risk during facelift surgery where the neck is fully undermined.

In the author's practice, the depth of resurfacing is determined by the anatomic location within the face or neck. The UltraPulse CO_2 laser (Lumenis) with the 1.3-mm spot size (ActiveFX) is used to treat both the face and upper neck. Treatment on the face typically ablates approximately two-thirds of the epidermis (depth of ablative injury is 80 μm) and thermally injures the remaining one-third of the epidermis. This protocol was developed specifically to fit the unique setting of treating undermined skin during facelift surgery. In the neck, however, this technique has been fully adopted as the standard treatment regimen regardless of surgical treatment to the neck. Energy settings are modified when treating the mid and lower neck below the first cervical crease to reflect the thinner epidermis and dermis. Density settings are also lowered to approximately 50% in consideration of the fewer adnexal structures present in this anatomic zone. Frequency settings are limited to 250 Hz. The author prefers to use a larger spot size with depth of penetration limited to the epidermis. (The 120-μm spot size available on the laser is typically used for deeper depth of injury not considered suitable for undermined neck skin.)

The resultant effect by the 1.3-mm superpulsed laser is that the epidermis experiences a combination of ablative and thermal injury at a depth that allows rapid healing. When the facelift (but not the neck lift) is completed, the laser treatment provides additional tightening, a shrink-wrap effect that enhances the effect of the facelift.

The author believes that treating the skin, or canvas, not only improves the appearance of the skin after facelift but also tightens the skin in ways that facelift surgery cannot. This additional skin contraction leads to a more natural appearing result by repairing and helping to recontour the facial skin. Because of the facial skin's more robust structure, specific areas within the face can be tailor tightened to enhance the surgical result. In the neck, however, the laser should not be used to achieve additional skin tightening.[47] Its treatment purpose should be to simply improve the appearance of the skin. The thin and more fragile skin in the neck does not tolerate the same aggressive resurfacing techniques that are possible on facial skin. Neck skin functions more like a canvas stretching over the platysma muscle, and attempts at aggressive resurfacing to tighten underlying structures are simply not prudent. Although clinical-histological correlation demonstrates that deeper penetration may result in more textural improvements,[55] deeper penetration into the reticular dermis may create wounds that are more difficult to heal, particularly when higher density levels are used.

Lasers that require multimillisecond pulse duration create significantly more thermal damage than lasers whose ablative threshold is less than 0.8 millisecond (see **Fig. 2**).[47] Hobbs and colleagues[56] demonstrated that if tissue heating occurs without vaporization, tissue temperatures may exceed 600°C, and residual thermal damage may be 300 μm to 1 mm or more, leading to poor wound healing and potential scarring. Despite the concept that ablative fractional lasers are safer than fully ablative lasers, the longer pulse width of a lower-energy fractional laser can create much more thermal damage when attempting to reach depths of 1000 μm, resulting in significant enough damage to delay wound healing and create scarring.[42,44] The upper and lower neck are treated differently. Because neck skin above the first cervical rhytid is similar to facial skin, the upper cervical neck skin can be treated similarly to facial skin. The lower two-thirds of neck, however, are approximately 40% thinner than skin above the first cervical crease and have fewer adnexal structures required for healing. The lower neck, therefore, requires different treatment settings to account for these anatomic and structural differences.[32,34] Currently, the author lowers the density to 50% (facial skin is treated at density greater than 90%) and removes approximately 75% of the epidermis by ablation and approximately 25% by thermal coagulation. The depth of injury reflects the epidermal depth of 70 μm and the papillary dermal depth of 60 μm.

Because the ultrapulsed laser delivers its ablative energy within 0.8 millisecond (0.8–1.0 millisecond is recognized as the thermal relaxation time [TRT] of human skin),[47] superheating or the propagation of increased thermal zones does not occur. This important concept must be taken into consideration if a health care provider is using a laser whose pulse width exceeds the TRT of skin. When the pulse width exceeds the TRT of skin, additional thermal effect occurs, resulting in increased density, wider zones of ablation, and even char formation with superheating below and adjacent to the target size. All of these phenomena can contribute to significant complications (shown in **Figs. 1** and **4**).[42,47]

Despite the belief by some investigators that ablative laser resurfacing of the neck may pose excessive risk in undermined skin, the author, during the past 5 years, has consistently resurfaced the upper and lower neck during facelift surgery to improve residual wrinkles and enhance tone and texture. Early treatments were limited to the upper neck skin above the first cervical crease, but it became evident that leaving the lower neck and décolletage untreated was unsatisfactory (**Fig. 5**).

By carefully applying the principles set forth by Anderson and Parrish[57] with regard to TRT, and using a device that is able to provide the necessary energy to ablate skin within the TRT of skin, consistent and safe results have been achieved in more than 400 facelift and neck lift patients. Clinical examples are shown in **Figs. 6** and **7**.

The author's choice to use a pulsed ablative CO_2 laser to rejuvenate skin was based on the gold standard status of the CO_2 laser and a novel

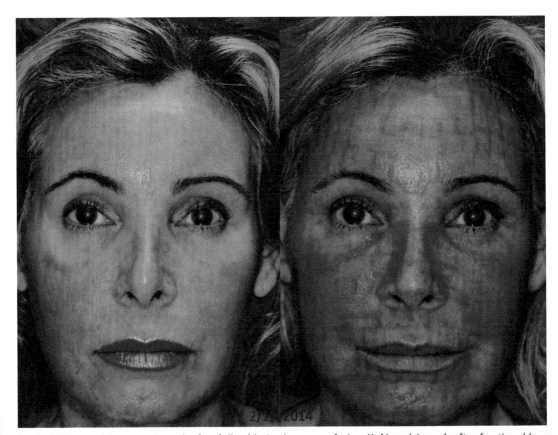

Fig. 4. A 56-year-old woman 1 week after fully ablative laser resurfacing (*left*) and 1 week after fractional laser resurfacing at 25% density and 450-μm depth (*right*). The fractional treatment was given 1 year after the ablative treatment. The ablative treatment removed the epidermis. Note the significant level of inflammation associated with the fractional treatment due to the prolonged pulse width associated with the depth of injury.

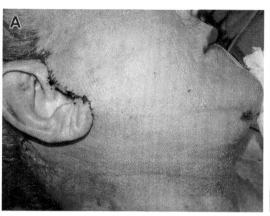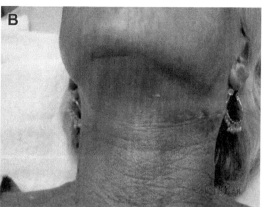

Fig. 5. (*A*) A side view of a 58-year-old woman after laser resurfacing of the face and upper cervical skin but not the lower neck and (*B*) an anterior view of the same patient 3 weeks after laser resurfacing. The untreated lower neck is unattractive compared with the noticeably improved upper neck.

post-treatment plan that greatly reduces adverse effects traditionally associated with fully ablative resurfacing. In this plan, a perfluorodecalin emulsion (Cutagenix, Cutagenesis) is applied after either fully ablative or fractional resurfacing reduces adverse effects traditionally associated with ablative resurfacing. Current postoperative care in the author's practice includes a shower twice daily and perfluorodecalin emulsion 3 times daily over treated areas. Continual use of cool compresses during healing helps to prevent dryness during the healing period. A detailed description of this post-treatment plan has recently become available.[47,58]

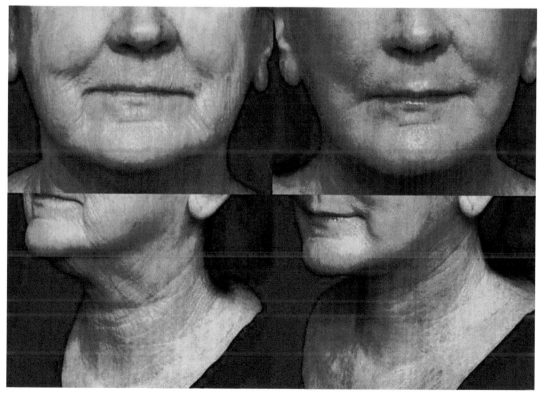

Fig. 6. Front and diagonal views of a 66-year-old woman before (*left*) and 3 months after a facelift and laser resurfacing of the face and neck by the author (*right*).

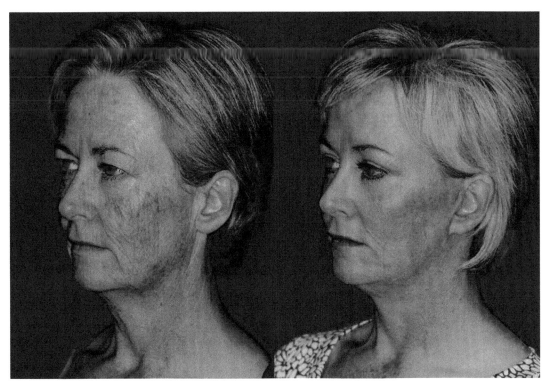

Fig. 7. Side views of a 54-year-old woman before (*left*) and after rejuvenation (*right*), which included fat grafting and laser resurfacing of face and neck. Note the lack of pigmentary changes on the resurfaced neck.

SUMMARY

The author currently performs CO_2 laser resurfacing with all facelift and neck lift surgeries and has found that these combinations provide predictable results when treatment parameters respect anatomic and physical properties of specific skin sites. The achievement of volume restoration, complete lifting, and skin rejuvenation together has provided high satisfaction rates among patients. Since the author has followed the perfluorodecalin emulsion protocol after laser treatment, hypopigmentation, scarring, and loss of skin have not been observed. The author does not, however, resurface undermined neck or facial skin with a deep fractional laser; resurfacing is limited to the epidermis. Although fully ablative superficial skin resurfacing does not provide the same results as facelift or neck surgery, the laser does provide a useful adjunct to neck surgery.

The use of the fully ablative, pulsed CO_2 laser as an adjunct to neck lift surgery, with or without facelift surgery, permits surgeons to fulfill the expectations of patients who want the skin of both their face and neck to be homogeneous and more attractive. The perfluorodecalin emulsion aftercare protocol reopens the case for using the fully ablative CO_2 laser to achieve the best possible resurfacing result. The risk of adverse effects is reduced simply by adjusting the treatment settings to take into account the reduced healing capacity of the neck compared with the face.

REFERENCES

1. Rohrich RJ, Rios JL, Smith PD, et al. Neck rejuvenation revisited. Plast Reconstr Surg 2006;118:1251–63.
2. Brandt FS, Boker A. Botulinum toxin for the treatment of neck lines and neck bands. Dermatol Clin 2004;22:159–66.
3. Goldman MP, Fitzpatrick RE, Manuskiatti W. Laser resurfacing of the neck with the Erbium:YAG laser. Dermatol Surg 1999;25:164–7 [discussion: 167–8].
4. Jimenez G, Spencer JM. Erbium:YAG laser resurfacing of the hands, arms, and neck. Dermatol Surg 1999;25:831–4 [discussion: 834–5].
5. Barton FE Jr. Aesthetic surgery of the face and neck. Aesthet Surg J 2009;29:449–63 [Erratum appears in Aesthet Surg J 2010;30:493].
6. Roy D. Neck rejuvenation. Dermatol Clin 2005;23: 469–74.
7. Alster TS, Konda S. Plasma skin resurfacing for regeneration of neck, chest, and hands: investigation of a novel device. Dermatol Surg 2007;33: 1315–21.

8. Matarasso A, Matarasso SL, Brandt FS, et al. Botulinum A exotoxin for the management of platysma bands. Plast Reconstr Surg 1999;103:645–52 [discussion: 653–5].

9. Kane MA. Nonsurgical treatment of platysmal bands with injection of botulinum toxin A. Plast Reconstr Surg 1999;103:656–63 [discussion: 664–5. Erratum appears in Plast Reconstr Surg 1999; 103:followi].

10. Carruthers J, Carruthers A. Aesthetic botulinum A toxin in the mid and lower face and neck. Dermatol Surg 2003;29:468–76.

11. Carruthers J, Carruthers A. Botulinum toxin A in the mid and lower face and neck. Dermatol Clin 2004; 22:151–8.

12. Manuskiatti W, Fitzpatrick RE, Goldman MP. Long-term effectiveness and side effects of carbon dioxide laser resurfacing for photoaged facial skin. J Am Acad Dermatol 1999;40:401–11.

13. Brody HJ. Complications of chemical peels. In: Brody HJ, editor. Chemical peeling. St Louis (MO): Mosby Yearbook; 1992.

14. Resnik SS, Resnik BI. Complications of chemical peeling. Dermatol Clin 1995;13:309–12.

15. Orentreich N, Orentreich DS. Dermabrasion. Dermatol Clin 1995;13:313–27.

16. Baker TJ, Gordon HL, Seckinger DL. A second look at chemical face peeling. Plast Reconstr Surg 1966;37:487–93.

17. Baker TJ, Gordon HL, Mosienko P, et al. Long-term histological study of skin after chemical face peeling. Plast Reconstr Surg 1974;53:522–5.

18. Kligman AM, Baker TJ, Gordon HL. Long-term histologic follow-up of phenol face peels. Plast Reconstr Surg 1985;75:652–9.

19. Benedetto AV, Griffin TD, Benedetto EA, et al. Dermabrasion: therapy and prophylaxis of the photoaged face. J Am Acad Dermatol 1992;27: 439–47.

20. Goldberg DJ, Meine JG. Treatment of photoaged neck skin with the pulsed Erbium:YAG laser. Dermatol Surg 1998;24:619–21.

21. Hetter GP. An examination of the phenol-croton oil peel: part I. Dissecting the formula. Plast Reconstr Surg 2000;105:227–39 [discussion: 249–51].

22. Hetter GP. An examination of the phenol croton oil peel: part II. The lay peelers and their croton oil formulas. Plast Reconstr Surg 2000;105:240–8 [discussion: 249–51. Erratum appears in Plast Reconstr Surg 2000;105:1083].

23. Hetter GP. An examination of the phenol-croton oil peel: part III. The plastic surgeons' role. Plast Reconstr Surg 2000;105:752–63.

24. Hetter GP. An examination of the phenol-croton oil peel: part IV. Face peel results with different concentrations of phenol and croton oil. Plast Reconstr Surg 2000;105:1061–83 [discussion: 1084–7].

25. Bensimon RH. Croton oil peels. Aesthet Surg J 2008;28:33–45 [Erratum appears in Aesthet Surg J 2008;28:221].

26. Baker TJ. Chemical face peeling and rhytidectomy. A combined approach for facial rejuvenation. Plast Reconstr Surg Transplant Bull 1962;29:199–207.

27. Bogle MA, Arndt KA, Dover JS. Evaluation of plasma skin regeneration technology in low-energy full-facial rejuvenation. Arch Dermatol 2007;143:168–74.

28. Alora MB, Anderson RR. Recent developments in cutaneous lasers. Lasers Surg Med 2000;26: 108–18.

29. Rox AR. Laser-tissue interactions. In: Goldman MP, editor. Cutaneous laser surgery. 2nd edition. St Louis (MO): Mosby; 1999.

30. Fanous N, Prinja N, Sawaf M. Laser resurfacing of the neck: a review of 48 cases. Aesthetic Plast Surg 1998;22:173–9.

31. Behroozan DS, Christian MM, Moy RL. Short-pulse carbon dioxide laser resurfacing of the neck. J Am Acad Dermatol 2000;43(1 Pt 1):72–6.

32. Fitzpatrick RE, Goldman MP, Sriprachya-Anunt S. Resurfacing of photodamaged skin on the neck with an UltraPulse((R)) carbon dioxide laser. Lasers Surg Med 2001;28:145–9.

33. Kilmer SL, Chotzen V, Zelickson BD, et al. Full-face laser resurfacing using a supplemented topical anesthesia protocol. Arch Dermatol 2003;139: 1279–83.

34. Rosenberg GJ. Full face and neck laser skin resurfacing. Plast Reconstr Surg 1997;100:1846–54.

35. Sasaki GH, Travis HM, Tucker B. Fractional CO2 laser resurfacing of photoaged facial and nonfacial skin: histologic and clinical results and side effects. J Cosmet Laser Ther 2009;11:190–201.

36. Goldman MP, Marchell NL. Laser resurfacing of the neck with the combined CO2/Er:YAG laser. Dermatol Surg 1999;25:923–5.

37. Weiss RA, Weiss MA, Beasley KL. Rejuvenation of photoaged skin: 5 years results with intense pulsed light of the face, neck, and chest. Dermatol Surg 2002;28:1115–9.

38. Dahan S, Lagarde JM, Turlier V, et al. Treatment of neck lines and forehead rhytids with a nonablative 1540 nm Er:glass laser: a controlled clinical study combined with the measurement of the thickness and the mechanical properties of the skin. Dermatol Surg 2004;30:872–9 [discussion: 879–80].

39. Tierney EP, Hanke CW. Ablative fractionated CO2, laser resurfacing for the neck: prospective study and review of the literature. J Drugs Dermatol 2009;8:723–31.

40. Manstein D, Herron GS, Sink RK, et al. Fractional photothermolysis: a new concept for cutaneous remodeling using microscopic patterns of thermal injury. Lasers Surg Med 2004;34:426–38.

41. Geronemus RG. Fractional photothermolysis: current and future applications. Lasers Surg Med 2006;38:169–76.

42. Avram MM, Tope WD, Yu T, et al. Hypertrophic scarring of the neck following ablative fractional carbon dioxide laser resurfacing. Lasers Surg Med 2009;41:185–8.

43. Shamsaldeen O, Peterson JD, Goldman MP. The adverse events of deep fractional CO(2): a retrospective study of 490 treatments in 374 patients. Lasers Surg Med 2011;43:453–6.

44. Fife DJ, Fitzpatrick RE, Zachary CB. Complications of fractional CO2 laser resurfacing: four cases. Lasers Surg Med 2009;41:179–84.

45. Walsh JT Jr, Flotte TJ, Anderson RR, et al. Pulsed CO2 laser tissue ablation: effect of tissue type and pulse duration on thermal damage. Lasers Surg Med 1988;8(2):108–18.

46. Ross EV, Domankevitz Y, Skrobal M, et al. Effects of CO2 laser pulse duration in ablation and residual thermal damage: implications for skin resurfacing. Lasers Surg Med 1996;19(2):123–9.

47. Duplechain JK. Fractional CO2 resurfacing: has it replaced ablative resurfacing techniques? Facial Plast Surg Clin North Am 2013;21:213–27.

48. Venugopalan V, Nishioka NS, Mikić BB. The effect of CO2 laser pulse repetition rate on tissue ablation rate and thermal damage. IEEE Trans Biomed Eng 1991;38:1049–52.

49. Bernstein LJ, Kauvar AN, Grossman MC, et al. The short- and long-term side effects of carbon dioxide laser resurfacing. Dermatol Surg 1997;23:519–25.

50. Nanni CA, Alster TS. Complications of carbon dioxide laser resurfacing. An evaluation of 500 patients. Dermatol Surg 1998;24:315–20.

51. Sriprachya-Anunt S, Fitzpatrick RE, Goldman MP, et al. Infections complicating pulsed carbon dioxide laser resurfacing for photoaged facial skin. Dermatol Surg 1997;23:527–35 [discussion: 535–6].

52. Schwartz RJ, Burns AJ, Rohrich RJ, et al. Long-term assessment of CO2 facial laser resurfacing: aesthetic results and complications. Plast Reconstr Surg 1999;103:592–601.

53. Berwald C, Levy JL, Magalon G. Complications of the resurfacing laser: retrospective study of 749 patients. Ann Chir Plast Esthet 2004;49:360–5.

54. Campbell TM, Goldman MP. Adverse events of fractionated carbon dioxide laser: review of 373 treatments. Dermatol Surg 2010;36:1645–50.

55. Tierney EP, Eisen RF, Hanke CW. Fractionated CO2 laser skin rejuvenation. Dermatol Ther 2011;24:41–53.

56. Hobbs ER, Bailin PL, Wheeland RG, et al. Super-pulsed lasers: minimizing thermal damage with short duration, high irradiance pulses. J Dermatol Surg Oncol 1987;13:955–64.

57. Anderson RR, Parrish JA. Selective photothermolysis: precise microsurgery by selective absorption of pulsed radiation. Science 1983;220:524–7.

58. Duplechain JK, Rubin MG, Kim K. Novel post-treatment care after ablative and fractional CO2 laser resurfacing. J Cosmet Laser Ther 2013. [Epub ahead of print].

Thermally Confined Micropulsed 1444-nm Nd:YAG Interstitial Fiber Laser in the Aging Face and Neck: An Update

J. David Holcomb, MD

KEYWORDS

- Laser • Lipolysis • Facial • Neck • Contouring • Facelift • Thermal confinement
- Thermal diffusivity

KEY POINTS

- The micropulsed 1444-nm Nd:YAG interstitial fiber laser enables precision contouring of the mid- and lower face and the neck, both as stand-alone procedures (laser-assisted facial contouring [LAFC] and laser-assisted neck contouring [LANC]) and as an adjunct during aging face surgery (laser-assisted facelift [LAFL]).
- Use of the 1444-nm Nd:YAG interstitial fiber laser requires knowledge regarding how to maintain safe clinical thermal confinement during treatment.
- Integrating this technology with facelift surgery facilitates elevation of (extended, if desired) cervicofacial rhytidectomy flaps, enables percutaneous release of major fascial retaining ligaments in the mid- and lower face, may obviate open submentoplasty and platysmaplasty in some patients, and facilitates greater posterior and superior repositioning of flaps for improved outcomes.

INTRODUCTION

Although the use of Nd:YAG fiber lasers in aesthetic surgery has been traditionally referred to as *laser lipolysis*, it is now evident that subcutaneous fat may not or need not be the primary laser target. As such, the use of Nd:YAG fiber lasers has evolved to include ablation and emulsification of subcutaneous fatty tissue, fibrolysis, and shrinkage of fine skin ligaments (ligamentae retinacula cutis) and more dense structural osseocutaneous anchoring ligaments (eg, zygomatic- and mandibular-cutaneous ligaments) as well as postulated direct tissue effects that may contribute to tightening of the skin and of the platysma muscle. Because the use of Nd:YAG fiber lasers goes beyond direct treatment of subcutaneous fat, some laser surgeons now advocate the term, *interstitial laser*, in lieu of laser lipolysis when referencing the use of these devices.

Subcutaneous Nd:YAG fiber laser tissue interaction is influenced by a variety of factors, including laser wavelength, power, pulse duration and total energy applied, target tissue composition, and relative amounts of exogenous water added to the treatment area. Collectively these factors influence opposing characteristics of fiber laser tissue interaction, termed *thermal confinement* and *thermal diffusivity* (discussed later), whereas related clinical implications affect subcutaneous Nd:YAG fiber laser treatment protocols and safety and immediately observed and late tissue effects.

Disclosure Statement: No current actual or potential conflict of interest, including employment, consultancies, stock ownership, patent applications/registrations, grants, and other funding.
Holcomb – Kreithen Plastic Surgery and MedSpa, 1 South School Avenue, Suite 800, Sarasota, FL 34237, USA
E-mail address: drholcomb@sarasota-med.com

Facial Plast Surg Clin N Am 22 (2014) 217–229
http://dx.doi.org/10.1016/j.fsc.2014.01.005
1064-7406/14/$ – see front matter © 2014 Elsevier Inc. All rights reserved.

Evaluation of absorption spectra for Nd:YAG fiber lasers reveals absorption in fat and water is greatest in the mid–1400-nm range, intermediate at 1320 nm, and least at 1064 nm.[1] The relative absorption is on the order of 1 magnitude higher for fat but many orders of magnitude higher for water In the mid–1400-nm range versus 1320 nm and 1064 nm.[1] A minor anhydrous collagen absorption peak present in the mid–1400-nm range may also influence laser energy absorption and laser tissue interaction.[2] Comparison of direct tissue effects reveals that fatty tissue ablation crater depth and fatty tissue ablation efficiency are greatest at 1444 nm, intermediate at 1320 nm, and least at 1064 nm.[2] Differences in tissue absorption and laser tissue interaction among Nd:YAG fiber lasers are summarized in **Table 1**.

Thermal confinement and thermal diffusivity are opposing characteristics of fiber laser tissue interaction that are of critical importance for exerting desired laser tissue effects while avoiding undesired complications. Thermal confinement refers to spatial limitation of tissue heating relatively near the tip of the laser fiber or more broadly within the desired tissue treatment area whereas thermal diffusivity refers to heat distribution away from the source or tip of the laser fiber via conduction.[2] Although the 2 phenomena are simultaneously present, the relative proportions are influenced by laser wavelength, power, and pulse duration as well as target tissue composition, tissue water content, and total laser energy applied to the treatment area—their differential effects on thermal confinement and diffusivity are summarized in **Table 2**.

Thermal imaging studies among the Nd:YAG fiber laser wavelengths demonstrate that thermal confinement is greatest at mid–1400 nm, intermediate at 1064 nm, and least at 1320 nm.[2] Clinically, improved thermal confinement translates to a longer lag period or larger therapeutic window that precedes significant heat accumulation in the larger laser treatment area. The ability of the tissue and exogenous water in the treatment area to maintain thermal confinement is exceeded at the far side of the therapeutic window where thermal diffusivity then prevails with more rapid tissue heating from that point forward. Various tissues have specific tolerances to prolonged heating—irreversible coagulation of the skin may occur with heating to 59°C for as little as 1 second.[3] Excessive thermal diffusion leading to irreversible tissue injury indicates a clinical failure of thermal confinement.

Native target tissue composition affects Nd:YAG fiber laser tissue interaction. Although relative adipocyte may not able to be estimated versus fibrous tissue content prior to laser treatment, this can be inferred based on the tissue response. If the tissues soften during treatment, significant fat emulsification and liquefaction have generally occurred. Significant firming and tightening of the tissues suggest a greater fibrous tissue content with contraction of collagen containing structures; significant fat emulsification and liquefaction may still have occurred despite the firmness but greater mechanical effort may be required for its removal during lipoaspiration.

INTERSTITIAL ND:YAG FIBER LASER–ASSISTED FACIAL CONTOURING

Interstitial Nd:YAG fiber LAFC may be used as a stand-alone percutaneous sculpting procedure for the midface, lower face/jawline, and the female round Asian face.[1] LAFC of the mid- and/or lower face as a stand-alone treatment is generally more successful in female patients. Volumetric sculpting of the mid- and/or lower face (ie, soft tissue reduction) with LAFC complements well-established procedures for soft tissue augmentation and enables synergy through a proportionally greater effect with soft tissue augmentation. Appropriate patient selection should include those with mild to moderate fullness and readily palpable subcutaneous fat but without excessive skin laxity. Patients with skin laxity but no significant subcutaneous fat are not appropriate candidates for the LAFC procedure. Patient age is not a major determining factor with regard to successful outcomes—very good LAFC results have been obtained with patients into their early 70s.

Table 1
Differences in tissue absorption and laser tissue interaction among Nd:YAG fiber lasers

	Mid–1400 nm	1320 nm	1064 nm
Water absorption	Highest[a]	Intermediate	Lowest
Fat absorption	Highest[a]	Intermediate	Lower
Collagen (anhydrous) absorption	Low[a]	—	—
Fatty tissue ablation efficiency	Highest	Intermediate	Least

[a] Absorption peaks for water, fat, and collagen occur in the mid–1400-nm range.

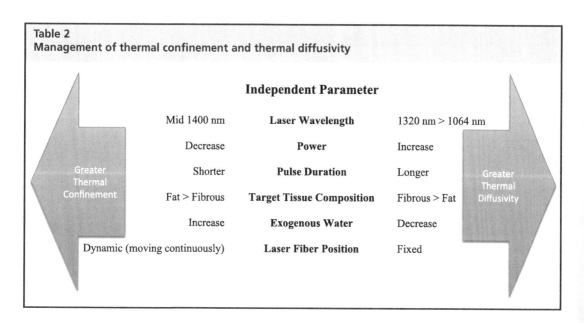

Table 2
Management of thermal confinement and thermal diffusivity

	Independent Parameter	
Mid 1400 nm	**Laser Wavelength**	1320 nm > 1064 nm
Decrease	**Power**	Increase
Shorter	**Pulse Duration**	Longer
Fat > Fibrous	**Target Tissue Composition**	Fibrous > Fat
Increase	**Exogenous Water**	Decrease
Dynamic (moving continuously)	**Laser Fiber Position**	Fixed

(Left arrow: Greater Thermal Confinement; Right arrow: Greater Thermal Diffusivity)

Mild to moderate post-treatment inflammatory edema (PIE) is expected. Early on, PIE seems to have blunted or limited the lower facial tissue contouring response; however, lower facial contour improves over time as PIE gradually resolves and the skin contracts. Early on (eg, weeks 2 through 6), weekly lymphatic massage sessions for the LAFC treatment areas may help reduce PIE and improve lower facial contour. Significant PIE may be treated with staged escalating-dose intralesional triamcinolone (eg, 10 mg/mL initially, gradually moving to 40 mg/mL) beginning at post-treatment month 1 or 2 and continuing monthly as needed until final desired contour is achieved or until no further tissue response. Although this approach is successful in a majority of patients with PIE, the origin of persistent lower facial fullness with palpable subcutaneous fullness in partial responders is not known.

Some of the adipocyte lipid content liberated during laser lipolysis may be subject to reuptake by adipocytes that remain at the periphery of the treatment area. A significant increase in body mass index after LAFC could also partially account for a blunted tissue response. It seems more likely, however, that the natural healing response to adipose tissue ischemia and adipocyte necrosis may stimulate a tissue regeneration response, with adipose tissue remodeling involving adjacent adipose-derived stem progenitor cells and formation of neoadipocytes—this phenomenon has been carefully elucidated in animal models for adipose tissue ischemia[4] and nonvascularized fat grafting.[5] Persistent fullness 6 to 12 months after

LAFC may be addressed through a touch-up percutaneous LAFC procedure.

LAFC treatment begins with identification and marking of the desired treatment areas. In keeping with anatomic studies of the jowl fat compartment,[6] the desired area of tissue ablation for contouring of the lower face and jawline may include subcutaneous tissue fullness at, below, and well above the caudal border of the mandible (**Fig. 1A**). In many patients, the position of the jowl changes substantially with supine or slight Trendelenburg positioning; therefore, patient marking for LAFC should be done with patients in an upright, seated position to most accurately ensure inclusion of the desired tissue in the outlined treatment areas. The LAFC percutaneous entry point should be at least 1.5-cm posterior to the posterior extent of the intended LAFC treatment zone to ensure that an adequate tissue seal is maintained between the entry point and the treatment zone. If the entry point is placed too close to the LAFC treatment zone, the lipoaspiration step may be more difficult and inefficient because air may easily be drawn into the aspiration syringe.

Ensuring that the desired tissue is treated during LAFC is accomplished via (1) minimizing any positional tissue shift with slight reverse Trendelenburg patient positioning (eg, 20°); (2) limiting exogenous water input with small amounts of local anesthetic used (eg, 3 mL); (3) using hyaluronidase to improve local anesthetic distribution through the tissues; and (4) isolating and stabilizing the target tissue between the user's thumb

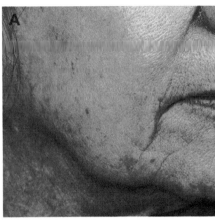 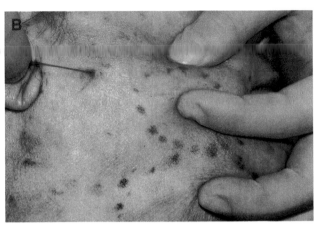

Fig. 1. (*A*) Preoperative view of LAFC treatment area with lower facial fullness and jowling in a 58-year-old woman in upright seated position. (*B*) Intraoperative view of LAFC treatment area in the same patient in 20° reverse Trendelenburg position. LAFC treatment zone is outlined with purple marker. LAFC entry site is located approximately 2 cm posterior to inked posterior extent of LAFC treatment zone and 2 cm above the caudal mandibular margin. The 600-μm bare laser fiber is present at the LAFC entry point and the red aiming beam at the fiber tip is seen faintly between the surgeon's gloved thumb and index finger. Note that the laser fiber is engaged in fatty tissue at the superior extent of the jowl fat compartment.

and forefinger during local anesthesia infiltration, laser energy delivery, and lipoaspiration. Limiting exogenous water infiltration to 3 mL minimizes distortion of the anatomy during treatment and facilitates endpoint identification but also limits thermal confinement. The fatty tissue ablation efficiency of the micropulsed 1444-nm Nd:YAG interstitial fiber laser, however, enables sufficient local tissue effect with preserved thermal confinement within the suggested total energy usage parameters.

The local anesthetic mixture that the author favors includes 0.5% lidocaine; 0.25% Bupivacaine hydrochloride; and 1:200,000 epinephrine and hyaluronidase, 2 to 4 IU per mL (eg, Hylenex recombinant, Halozyme Therapeutics, San Diego, CA, USA). Initially, approximately 1.0 mL of this local anesthetic mixture is used to provide anesthesia to the percutaneous entry site and the intervening tissue toward the LAFC treatment zone as well as a field block that includes the tissue for debulking and contouring. A narrow (eg, 21-gauge) multihole infiltration cannula is then used to deliver 3 mL of local anesthetic to the LAFC treatment area.

With the thermally confined micropulsed 1444-nm Nd:YAG interstitial fiber laser, energy delivery occurs via a 600-μm silica multimode fiber with the fiber used either free (bare) or assembled with a disposable or nondisposable cannula. Prior studies have demonstrated general safety guidelines for energy delivery during LAFC of the lower face when using the micropulsed 1444-nm Nd:YAG interstitial fiber laser and minimal volume

local anesthesia (dry technique)—typical parameters include power 5.4 W, pulse energy 180 mJ, pulse duration 100 μs (fixed), pulse rate 30 Hz, and total energy delivered 200 to 300 J.[1,7]

Although the unique thermal signature of the micropulsed 1444-nm Nd:YAG interstitial fiber laser enables safe treatment without the need for internal or external temperature monitoring, it is important to keep the fiber continuously moving through the tissue during active lasing—this facilitates even distribution of laser energy and limits the potential for clinical thermal confinement failure. Certainly some latitude exists with regard to these treatment parameters; however, in a prior study of mid- and lower face LAFC, complications, such as prolonged inflammatory edema and overcorrection, were associated with faster energy delivery (40 Hz) and with a doubling of the total energy delivered (eg, 500 J).[1] Immediately after energy delivery, a similar volume (eg, 3 mL) of room temperature sterile saline is infiltrated into the treatment area as a postcooling or thermal quenching step that attempts to minimize collateral thermal spread to adjacent tissues as well as reduce PIE.

Removal of emulsified tissue and liquefied fat via manual lipoaspiration with a small dual port aspiration cannula (eg, 19 gauge) and a 6-mL syringe (prefilled with 1-mL sterile saline) enables definitive tissue contouring. **Fig. 2** shows the full minimal instrumentation requirement for LAFC. It is not uncommon for a small-diameter aspiration cannula to become blocked with fibrous tissue during lipoaspiration—when this occurs, the cannula is

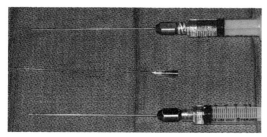

Fig. 2. LAFC instrumentation. (*Top*) 21-Gauge multi-hole infiltration cannula attached to 6-mL syringe containing 3-mL local anesthetic solution. (*Middle*) 600-μm Bare laser fiber with red diode aiming beam visible (*left*) and 18-gauge needle (*right*). (*Bottom*) 19-Gauge dual port aspiration cannula attached to 6-mL syringe prefilled with 1.0-mL sterile saline.

detached and irrigated until clear and then reattached to the same syringe and the procedure continued. If the syringe becomes filled with air, the seal at the syringe hub may need to be tightened or the percutaneous entry point may be too close to the treatment area. If the latter is the case, the procedure can usually continue with gentle manual occlusive pressure placed over the entry point area. Any air in the syringe can be gently expelled but with care to not also expel any fat already aspirated at this point. At the end of the lipoaspiration, the fat aspirate volume (less 1.0 mL from sterile saline prefilling) from each side is recorded in the treatment record. Mean volumes removed during unilateral lower face LAFC treatment approximate 2.5 mL in 2 studies, with ranges extending from 0.5 mL to more than 5.0 mL.[1,7] **Table 3** outlines major LAFC treatment steps and typical treatment parameters.

Initially, the aspiration cannula should be more superficial (immediately subcutaneous), with ports directed down. Effective debulking in areas of maximal subcutaneous tissue thickness, however, generally requires guiding the cannula into these areas at a deeper level. Although contrary to what has been an accepted tenet for traditional cold liposuction techniques, it is permissible and often helpful to remove some of the immediately subcutaneous fatty tissue adherent to the undersurface of the skin by using the lipoaspiration cannula with the ports directed upward toward the undersurface of the dermis. It is the author's belief that failure to do so may limit the facial contour, related skin contraction, and the ultimate result obtained.

Immediately after treatment, a compression dressing is applied that consists of 1 or 2 layers of 1-inch–thick roll cotton and a compression garment (eg, Universal Facial Band, Design Veronique, Richmond, CA, USA). The wound is evaluated the next day and the cotton is removed but patients are encouraged to wear the compression garment as much as possible for at least 1 week after treatment. Patient expectations must be carefully managed during the recovery and extended post-treatment period (as described previously). **Fig. 3** depicts before and long-term (>2 years) clinical photography following LAFC of the mid- and lower face as well as laser-assisted neck contouring.

INTERSTITIAL ND:YAG FIBER LASER–ASSISTED NECK CONTOURING

Interstitial Nd:YAG fiber LANC may be performed as a stand-alone percutaneous neck contouring procedure. Appropriate patient selection should include those with mild to moderate fullness in the submentum and neck with accumulated subcutaneous fatty tissue in these areas but without excessive skin laxity. Patients with skin laxity but

Table 3	
Major LAFC treatment steps and typical treatment parameters	
LAFC Treatment Step	**Detailed Information**
Field block[a]	Include percutaneous access point and target tissue
Infiltrate target tissue[a]	3 mL each LAFC treatment area (21-gauge multihole infiltration cannula)
Apply laser energy	Up to 200 J midface; up to 400 J for jawline Typical laser treatment parameters 5.4 W, 180 mJ, 30 Hz
Postcooling (thermal quenching)	Infiltrate 3-mL room temperature sterile saline (21-gauge multihole infiltration cannula)
Aspiration	Mean 2.5 mL (19-gauge dual port aspiration cannula attached to 6-mL syringe prefilled with 1.0-mL saline)
Compression	Roll cotton and elastic compression garment

[a] Local anesthetic mixture contains 0.5% lidocaine, 0.25% Bupivacaine hydrochloride, 1:200,000 epinephrine, and 2 IU hyaluronidase per mL.

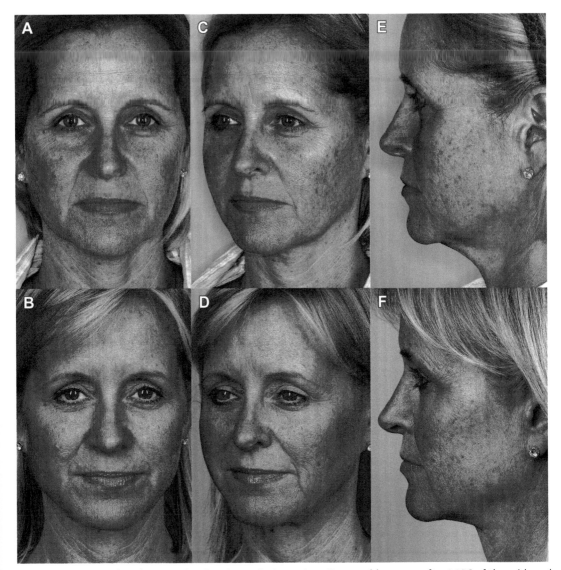

Fig. 3. Before (*A*, *C*, *E*) and 25 months after (*B*, *D*, *F*) photos in a 49-year-old woman after LAFC of the mid- and lower face and LANC (percutaneous). Treatment parameters for the mid- and lower face included 3.0 mL local/tumescent anesthetic, laser power 5.4 W, treatment speed 30 Hz, pulse energy 180 mJ, total energy delivered 400 J and 1.0- to 1.5-mL lipoaspirate. Treatment parameters for the submentum included 12.0-mL local/tumescent anesthetic, laser power 8.0 W, treatment speed 40 Hz, pulse energy 200 mJ, total energy delivered 1000 J and 5.0-mL lipoaspirate.

no significant subcutaneous fat are not appropriate candidates for the LANC procedure. Patient age is not a major determining factor with regard to successful outcomes—very good LANC results have been obtained with patients into their late 60s.

Mild to moderate PIE is expected. Early on PIE seems to have blunted or limited the submental/neck tissue contouring response; however, the tissue contour and cervicomental angle improve over time as PIE gradually resolves and the skin

contracts. Early on (eg, weeks 2 through 6), weekly lymphatic massage sessions for the LANC treatment area may help reduce PIE and improve submentum/neck contour. Significant PIE may be treated with staged escalating-dose intralesional triamcinolone (eg, 10 mg/mL initially, gradually moving to 40 mg/mL) beginning at post-treatment month 1 or 2 and continuing monthly as needed until final desired contour is achieved or until no further tissue response is seen. Although this approach is successful in a majority of patients with PIE, the cause of persistent full-ness with palpable subcutaneous fullness in partial responders is not known but similar mechanisms may be inferred in both the lower face and neck. Persistent fullness 6 to 12 months after LANC treatment may be addressed through a touch-up percutaneous LANC procedure.

LANC treatment begins with identification and marking of the treatment area. Although patient positioning does not affect the submentum and neck soft tissues as dramatically as in the lower face, marking for LANC is conventionally done with patients in an upright, seated position to most accurately ensure inclusion of the desired tissue in the outlined treatment area. Depending on body habitus, the treatment zone may extend laterally well into the central and toward the posterior aspect of level I in the neck as well as inferiorly to or well beyond the thyroid prominence in the anterior neck. In most patients, the LANC percutaneous entry point is conveniently placed at or just above the submental skin crease.

Ensuring that the desired tissue is treated during LANC is accomplished via the following steps: (1) limiting exogenous water input with small amounts of local anesthetic used (eg, 12–24 mL); (2) using hyaluronidase to improve local anesthetic distribution through the tissues; and (3) isolating and stabilizing the target tissue between the user's thumb and forefinger during local anesthesia infiltration, laser energy delivery, and lipoaspiration. Limiting exogenous water infiltration to approximately 12 mL minimizes distortion of the anatomy during treatment, facilitates endpoint identification, and limits thermal confinement. The fatty tissue ablation efficiency of the micropulsed 1444-nm Nd:YAG interstitial fiber laser, however, enables an adequate local tissue effect with preserved thermal confinement within the total energy usage parameters suggested. The local anesthetic mixture that the author favors for the submentum and neck includes 0.25% lidocaine, 0.125% Bupivacaine hydrochloride, 1:400,000 epinephrine, and hyaluronidase 1 to 2 IU per mL (eg, Hylenex recombinant). Initially, approximately 2.0 mL of this local anesthetic mixture is used to provide anesthesia to the percutaneous entry site as well as a field block that includes the tissue for debulking and contouring. A 1.6-mm multihole infiltration cannula (Tulip Medical Products, San Diego, CA, USA) is then used to deliver the local anesthetic to the LANC treatment area.

As in the lower face, the thermally confined micropulsed 1444-nm Nd:YAG interstitial fiber laser energy delivery occurs via a 600-μm silica multimode fiber with the fiber used either free (bare) or assembled with a disposable or nondisposable cannula. Prior studies have demonstrated general safety guidelines for energy delivery during LANC when using the micropulsed 1444-nm Nd:YAG interstitial fiber laser and minimal volume local anesthesia (dry technique)—typical parameters include power 8.0 to 10.0 W, pulse energy 200 to 250 mJ, pulse duration 100 μs (fixed), pulse rate 40 Hz, and total energy delivered 750 to 2000 J.[7] The mean total energy delivery for LANC in a cohort of approximately 180 neck contouring patients was just over 950 J whereas mean local anesthesia infiltration and lipoaspiration volumes were approximately 12.5 mL each in this same group.[7] **Table 4** outlines major LANC treatment steps and typical treatment parameters.

Because the neck skin is thinner (than in the lower face) and the energy delivery parameters are higher (than in LAFC), it is even more important to keep the fiber continuously moving through the

---

Table 4
Major LANC treatment steps and typical treatment parameters

LANC Treatment Step	Detailed Information
Field block[a]	Include percutaneous access point and target tissue
Infiltrate target tissue[a]	12–24 (mean 12.5) mL each LAFC treatment area using Tulip 1.6-mm multihole infiltration cannula
Apply laser energy	1000 (+) J Typical laser parameters 8.0–10.0 W, 200–250 mJ, 40 Hz
Postcooling (thermal quenching)	Infiltrate 12-mL room temperature sterile saline (Tulip 1.6-mm multihole infiltration cannula)
Aspiration	Mean 12.5 mL (Tulip 2.1-mm offset triple port aspiration cannula attached to 12 mL syringe prefilled with 1.0-mL saline)
Compression	Roll cotton and elastic compression garment

[a] Local anesthetic mixture contains 0.25% lidocaine, 0.125% Bupivacaine hydrochloride, 1:400,000 epinephrine, and 1 IU hyaluronidase per mL.

tissue while actively lasing during LANC—this facilitates even distribution of laser energy and limits the potential for clinical thermal confinement failure. Some latitude exists with regard to energy delivery and treatment parameters but the author suggests that surgeons proceed with caution with energy delivery totals exceeding 1000 J during LANC with these settings. At higher total energy delivery settings, the neck skin may become slightly to noticeably warm. Immediately after energy delivery, a similar volume (eg, 12 mL) of room temperature sterile saline is infiltrated into the treatment area.

Removal of emulsified tissue and liquefied fat via manual lipoaspiration with a 2.1-mm offset triple port aspiration cannula (Tulip) and a 12-mL syringe (prefilled with 1-mL sterile saline) enables definitive tissue contouring. **Fig. 4** depicts the full minimal instrumentation requirement for LANC. Use of the Tulip Snap Lok facilitates efficient lipoaspiration while allowing a surgeon to focus on tissue contouring. As with performing LAFC, the aspiration cannula may well become blocked during lipoaspiration, so the blockage must be cleared, as discussed previously, and the procedure continued. If the syringe becomes filled with air, then the same remedies can be applied as described previously, taking care not to expel any fat already aspirated at this point. At the end of the lipoaspiration, the fat aspirate volume (less 1.0 mL from sterile saline prefilling) is recorded in the treatment record.

Initially, the aspiration cannula should be more superficial (immediately subcutaneous) with the ports directed down. Effective debulking in areas of maximal subcutaneous tissue thickness, however, generally requires guiding the cannula into these areas at a deeper level. Using a gentle technique, it is helpful to remove some of the

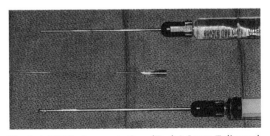

Fig. 4. LANC instrumentation. (*Top*) 1.6-mm Tulip multihole infiltration cannula attached to 12-mL syringe containing local anesthetic solution. (*Middle*) 60-μm Bare laser fiber with red diode aiming beam visible (*left*) and 18-gauge needle (*right*). (*Bottom*) 2.1-mm Tulip triple port (ports offset or nonaxial with only 1 port showing) aspiration cannula attached to 12-mL syringe prefilled with 1.0-mL sterile saline (Tulip Snap Lok not shown).

immediately subcutaneous fatty tissue adherent to the undersurface of the skin by using the lipoaspiration cannula with the ports directed upward toward the undersurface of the dermis. Generally a yellow or orange emulsion of subcutaneous fatty tissue is obtained. Depending on the volume of lipoaspirate, a second syringe may be needed to complete the procedure. The lipoaspiration portion of the procedure concludes when the desired tissue contour is achieved or when the emulsified fat aspirate return wanes or becomes blood tinged.

Persistent dermal to platysma fibrous attachments may represent a potential limiting factor with regard to the ability of the neck skin to adequately contract. After the lipoaspirate is obtained, the cannula is used in a sweeping motion to manually avulse any remaining fibrous attachments that may limit appropriate repositioning of the skin. Occasionally it may be necessary to transition the percutaneous LANC procedure to an open LANC procedure. If significant submental fullness is still evident, then a submental incision may be needed for direct evaluation for platysma muscle laxity and ptosis, bulky fat adherent to undersurface of the skin flap, and excess subplatysmal fatty tissue—if present, these findings are addressed surgically.

Immediately after treatment, a compression dressing is applied in a similar manner as for post-LAFC with a layer or 2 of thick cotton and a compression garment. The wound is evaluated the next day and the cotton is removed, but patients are encouraged to wear the compression garment as much as possible for at least 1 week after treatment. Patient expectations must be carefully managed during the recovery and extended post-treatment period, as described previously. **Fig. 5** shows interim results (3 months) in a patient with substantial submental fullness and skin laxity.

INTERSTITIAL ND:YAG FIBER LASER–ASSISTED FACE AND NECK LIFT—TREATMENT METHOD

Adjunctive use of the thermally confined micropulsed 1444-nm Nd:YAG interstitial fiber laser during face and neck lift surgery involves incorporation of the LAFC and LANC procedures where indicated with additional use of the laser for development of skin flaps and for lysis of osseocutaneous anchoring ligaments in the mid- and lower face. It should be appreciated that the jowl may encompass a significant volume of tissue above and below (with aging) the caudal margin of the mandible and that the jowl position may change significantly with patient positioning for facial

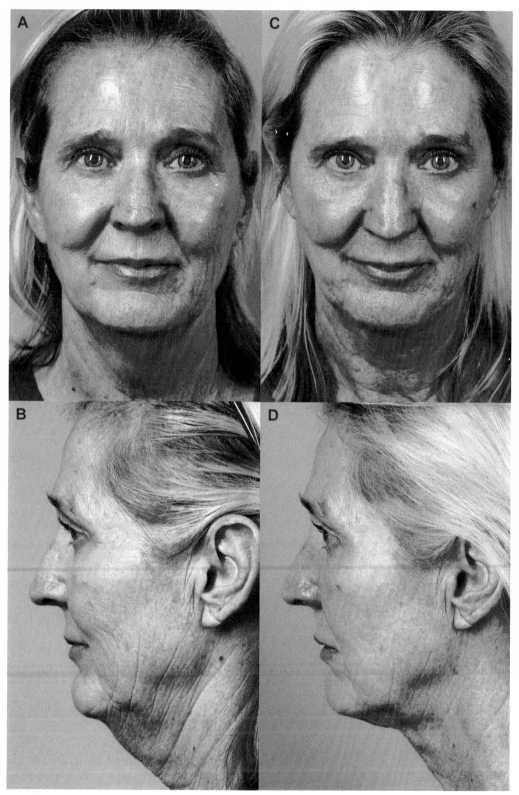

Fig. 5. Before (*A*, *C*) and after (*B*, *D*) photos in a 58-year-old woman 3 months after LANC (percutaneous). Treatment parameters included 18.0-mL local/tumescent anesthetic, laser power 10.0 W, treatment speed 40 Hz, pulse energy 250 mJ, total energy delivered 2000 J, and 20.0-mL lipoaspirate.

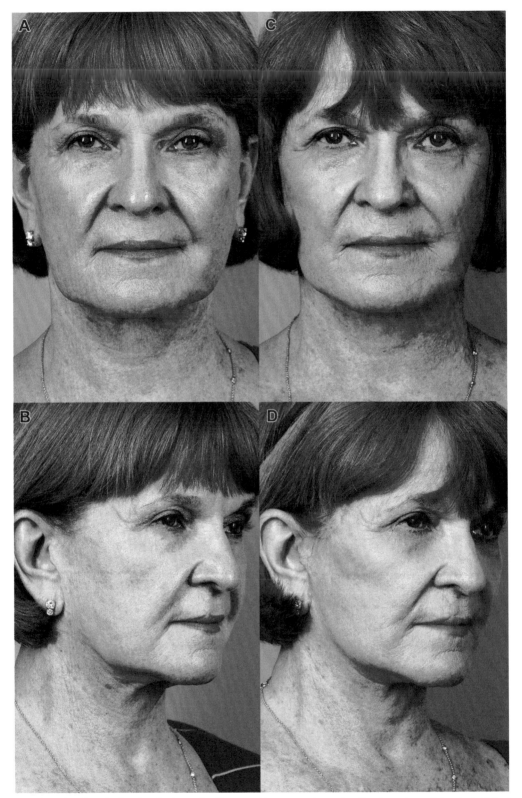

Fig. 6. Before (*A, C*) and after (*B, D*) photos in 67-year-old woman 1 month after temple and cheek rhytidectomy tuck with LAFC of the mid- and lower face and LANC (percutaneous). Treatment parameters for the mid- and lower face included 2.0- to 3.0-mL local anesthetic, laser power 5.4 W, treatment speed 30 Hz, pulse energy 180 mJ, total energy delivered 200 to 300 J, and 1.0- to 2.0-mL lipoaspirate. LANC treatment parameters included 12.0-mL local/ tumescent anesthetic, laser power 5.4 W, treatment speed 30 Hz, pulse energy 180 mJ, total energy delivered 150 J, and 5.0-mL lipoaspirate.

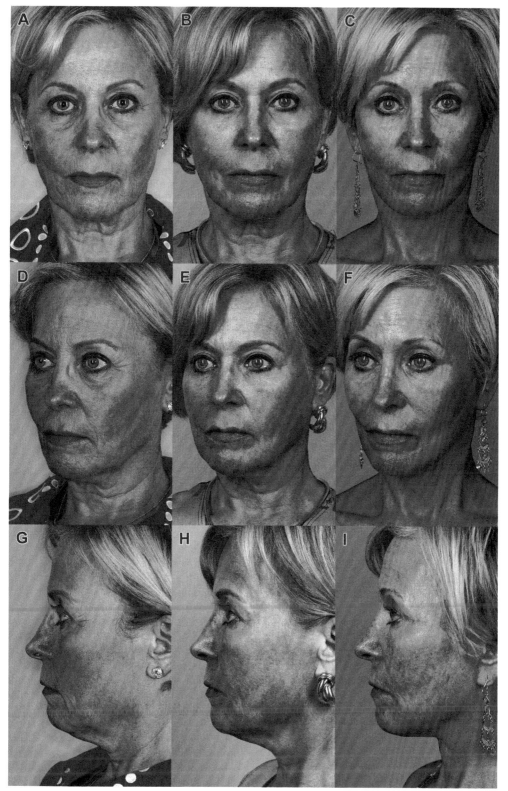

Fig. 7. Before (*A–C*), 6 months after LAFC mid- and lower face with autologous fat grafting and full face CO_2 ablative fractional resurfacing (*D–F*), and then 10 months after LAFL with LANC (percutaneous, converted to open approach but without platysmaplasty) and upper eyelid blepharoplasty (*G–I*) photos in a 59-year-old woman. Treatment parameters for the mid- and lower face included 2.0-mL local anesthetic, laser power 5.4 W, treatment speed 30 Hz, pulse energy 180 mJ, total energy delivered 150 J, and 1.0 to 2.0 mL lipoaspirate. LANC treatment parameters included 10.0-mL local/tumescent anesthetic, laser power 8.0 W, treatment speed 40 Hz, pulse energy 200 mJ, total energy delivered 1000 J, and 11.0-mL lipoaspirate.

surgery. The outline of the jowl may be readily evident with the patient in the upright, seated position for preoperative marking; however, due to tissue laxity and the effect of gravity, the marked tissue slated for contouring and debulking may move both superiorly and posteriorly when a patient is placed in the supine or Trendelenburg position for facial surgery.[7]

Ensuring adequate lower facial contouring may be accomplished by minimizing any positional tissue shift with a slight reverse Trendelenburg patient positioning (eg, 20°) and by isolating and stabilizing the target tissue between the user's thumb and forefinger during local anesthesia infiltration, laser energy delivery, and lipoaspiration. It may be, nonetheless, initially surprising to laser surgeons that the lower face LAFC procedure may involve contouring tissue a significant distance above the caudal margin of the mandible in some patients (see **Fig. 1**B). The central submental and neck tissue is less affected by patient positioning but adequate contouring in this area also requires manual guiding of the laser fiber into the areas of tissue fullness.

Although LANC enables a closed (percutaneous) approach to the neck in some facelift patients, persistent submental fullness and/or significant skin laxity immediately after LANC are indications for converting the initially closed procedure to an open procedure via a submental crease incision. Through this greater access, the effects of the LANC procedure may be assessed and any required surgical intervention (eg, midline imbrication platysmaplasty) may be performed. A recent study suggests that even though a converted open approach may be ideal, in many cases, surgical manipulation of the platysma may be required in only 20% of cases.[7] In cases of excess skin laxity, retrograde dissection at the lateral margins of the LANC treatment area, including subdermal release of the mandibular cutaneous ligament, may be performed via scissor dissection or laser fibrolysis.

The laser may be used to initiate the posterior cervicofacial skin flap dissection via fibrolysis and shrinkage of fine skin ligaments as well as for subdermal release of the zygomatic-cutaneous ligament. Safety of the skin flaps certainly takes precedence over use of the laser for this purpose. With appropriate treatment settings, limits on total energy applied, and proper technique, this application does not require anything other than the normal local anesthetic injection technique. Typical parameters that the author used for laser flap predissection include power 5.4 W, pulse energy 180 mJ, pulse duration 100 μs (fixed), pulse rate 30 Hz, and total energy delivered 200 to 300 J. Even

delivery of laser energy at the subdermal level throughout the flap minimizes the risk of a skin flap complication. Laser flap predissection decreases the subsequent physical effort and time required to complete the flap elevation with facelift scissors. With these treatment parameters, bleeding from some vascular perforators, both on the flap and the underlying tissue, requires bipolar cautery for hemostasis.

Laser flap predissection should include subdermal release of the zygomatic-cutaneous ligament as well as connecting the posterior cervicofacial dissection with the LAFC and LANC treatment areas. Fully coalescing the LAFC and LANC treatment areas with the posterior cervicofacial dissection enables greater posterior and vertical repositioning of the skin flaps but also requires more effective management of the skin flaps to harness the potential for improved outcomes.[7] **Figs. 6** and **7** demonstrate how the LAFC and LANC techniques may be integrated into aging face surgery to enhance outcomes.

SUMMARY

Integration of the thermally confined, micropulsed 1444-nm Nd:YAG interstitial fiber laser into minimally invasive and surgical management of the aging face and neck provides numerous benefits and some additional treatment options that are helpful for optimization of the 3-D contours of the mid- and lower face and neck. Currently LAFC may be the best nonsurgical answer to the main limitation faced by soft tissue augmentation (ie, that it does not address adjacent areas of soft tissue fullness). As such, one-sided attempts to enhance the appearance of the face with soft tissue augmentation may result in exaggerated features and excess fullness in attempting to camouflage descended fat in the mid- and lower face. Even subtle soft tissue debulking with LAFC improves the effective proportional enhancement of soft tissue augmentation.

LANC is an effective stand-alone percutaneous procedure for mild to moderate submental and neck soft tissue excess and skin laxity. The LAFL approach expands the use of this Nd:YAG interstitial fiber laser beyond LAFC and LANC to predissection of surgical flaps and release of osseocutaneous anchoring ligaments while also raising the possibility for percutaneous (closed) treatment of the neck and the platysma.

REFERENCES

1. Holcomb JD, Turk J, Baek SJ, et al. Laser-assisted facial contouring using a thermally confined

1444-nm Nd-YAG laser: a new paradigm for facial sculpting and rejuvenation. Facial Plast Surg 2011; 27(4):315–30.

2. Youn JI, Holcomb JD. Ablation efficiency and relative thermal confinement measurements using wavelengths 1,064, 1,320, and 1,444 nm for laser-assisted lipolysis. Lasers Med Sci 2013; 28(2):519–27.

3. Berlien HP, Muller GJ, editors. Applied laser medicine. Berlin: Springer; 2003.

4. Suga H, Eto H, Aoi N, et al. Adipose tissue remodeling under ischemia: death of adipocytes and activation of stem/progenitor cells. Plast Reconstr Surg 2010;126(6):1911–23.

5. Eto H, Kato H, Suga H, et al. The fate of adipocytes after nonvascularized fat grafting: evidence of early death and replacement of adipocytes. Plast Reconstr Surg 2012;129(5):1081–92.

6. Rohrich RJ, Pessa JE. The fat compartments of the face: anatomy and clinical implications for cosmetic surgery. Plast Reconstr Surg 2007;119(7): 2219–27.

7. Holcomb JD. Laser assisted facelift. Facial Plastic Surg, in press.

Adjunctive Procedures to Neck Rejuvenation

Mark M. Hamilton, MD[a,b,*], David Chan, MD[a]

KEYWORDS

- Neck rejuvenation • ARTISS • Fibrin sealant • Chin augmentation • Submandibular gland ptosis

KEY POINTS

- Chin projection should be evaluated in all patients seeking neck rejuvenation, and augmentation offered if indicated.
- Treatment of enlarged or ptotic submandibular glands is more invasive and carries with it significant risks, but is feasible.
- Fibrin sealants remove the need for drains postoperatively and help to improve the overall surgical experience.

INTRODUCTION

Rejuvenation of the neck often requires more than just a neck lift. A variety of steps and procedures exist to enhance the surgical technique or the overall result. Fibrin sealants can be used to improve the recovery process and are well documented in several recent studies.[1,2] Chin augmentation can be a critical part of creating a more refined neckline. Other procedures, such as submandibular gland excision, have been put forth by some as helpful to the overall aesthetic result. The position of the hyoid bone also plays an important role in the overall appearance of the neck. This article focuses on techniques beyond lifting and resurfacing that may enhance rejuvenation of the neck.

FIBRIN SEALANTS

The standard lifting techniques for the neck (neck lift, lower rhytidectomy) typically require the presence of drains after surgery. Elevation of facial flaps creates a dead space. Drains are used to remove fluid and blood that can collect below the flaps after surgery. Drains, however, are a nuisance for patients and their families, requiring instruction and care. Many patients are reluctant to have surgery because of fear or concern regarding drains. In addition, drains have been associated with infection, pain, and vessel and nerve injury. During consultation before and after surgery, many patients express dissatisfaction with the need for drains.

Fibrin sealants have been introduced in hopes of avoiding the requirement for drains and to improve the recovery process. Fibrin sealants have been used for decades in a variety of medical applications. The fibrin sealant consists of human fibrinogen, human thrombin, and bovine aprotinin. When these are mixed, they stimulate clot formation and the final phase of coagulation (**Fig. 1**). Continuation of this process forms a stronger clot, with a fully formed fibrin network. This is thought to enhance the healing process and seal capillaries, reducing oozing and bleeding. Studies have shown that fibrin sealants are able to enhance adherence of tissues to the wound bed.[3] What benefits come from that is a more controversial subject.

Disclosures: None.
[a] Department of Otolaryngology – Head and Neck Surgery, Indiana University School of Medicine, Indianapolis, IN, USA; [b] Hamilton Facial Plastic Surgery, 533 East County Line Road, Suite #104, Greenwood, IN 46143, USA
* Corresponding author. Hamilton Facial Plastic Surgery, 533 East County Line Road, Suite #104, Greenwood, IN 46143.
E-mail address: mmckhamilton@gmail.com

Facial Plast Surg Clin N Am 22 (2014) 231–242
http://dx.doi.org/10.1016/j.fsc.2014.01.008
1064-7406/14/$ – see front matter © 2014 Elsevier Inc. All rights reserved.

facialplastic.theclinics.com

Coagulation Cascade: Key Final Steps

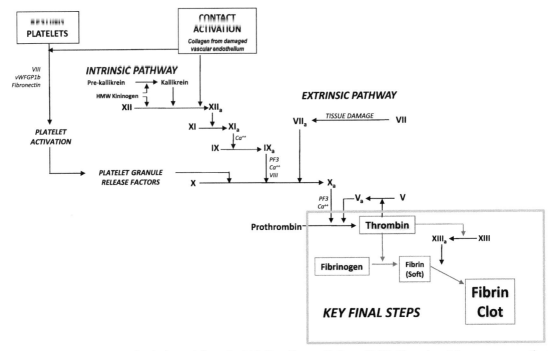

Fig. 1. Coagulation cascade. (*Adapted from* Oz MC, Rondinone JF, Shargill NS. Floseal matrix: new generation topical hemostatic sealant. J Card Surg 2003;18:486–93; with permission.)

The first reported use of fibrin glue in facial plastic surgery was by Ellis in 1988.[4] TISSEEL (Baxter Healthcare Corp, Deerfield, IL) was used in a variety of general ear, nose, and throat and facial plastic procedures. As for cosmetic procedures, TISSEEL was felt to be most beneficial in blepharoplasties and facelifts. Ellis noted that although it was no substitute for good surgical technique and maintenance of hemostasis, it was useful in minimizing venous bleeding, oozing, and even tiny capillary arterial bleeding.

Multiple studies followed Ellis' account, some reporting significant benefits, others less so. One consistent theme noted is the reduction in drain output with the use of fibrin sealants. This was noted by Oliver and colleagues[5] in a prospective, randomized, double-blind trial of the use of fibrin sealants in facelifts. Other studies have followed with TISSEEL and other fibrin sealants that have showed similar findings.[1,2,6] It is thought by many that with less drainage, the need for drains is reduced if not eliminated.

What remains a question is if fibrin sealants are helpful in reducing hematomas, seromas, bruising, swelling, and the recovery process in general. Several good studies have shown benefit, whereas others less so. Zoumalan and Rizk[7] found that patients undergoing rhytidectomy treated

with fibrin glue and no drains had a lower rate of hematomas than those who had the placement of drains. Similarly, Fezza and colleagues[8] noted patients undergoing rhytidectomy with fibrin sealants had less bruising and swelling and no hematomas. Other studies, such as that by Powell and colleagues,[9] showed positive trends with fibrin sealants, but no statistically significant benefit. Probably most telling of the controversy is the reported experience of Marchac and colleagues.[10,11] In 1994, Marchac and Sandor[10] reported a reduced rate of hematoma formation in a large series of patients undergoing rhytidectomy with fibrin sealants, but no drains or dressing. In addition, less bruising and swelling were noted in the group receiving fibrin sealants. A decade later, Marchac and Greensmith[11] concluded the theoretical benefit of fibrin sealants was not as great as they had hoped. This second study of 30 consecutive patients showed no difference in bruising, swelling, drain output, or hematoma incidence.[11]

Our experience with fibrin sealants has been with ARTISS (Baxter Healthcare Corp), which is a human-derived fibrin sealant. It received approval from the Food and Drug Administration (FDA) in 2008 for use in adhering autologous skin grafts to surgically prepared wound beds resulting from burns. It differs from TISSEEL in that it has a lower concentration of thrombin (4 IU/mL vs 500 IU/mL), allowing more time for tissue flap positioning. Typically the surgeon has about 60 seconds to prepare and position the flap before polymerization, and thus adherence, begins.

ARTISS received FDA approval as a fibrin sealant for facelift procedures in 2012. Studies for FDA approval showed that although ARTISS reduced drainage volume when used with facelifts, it provided no statistically significant reduction in the incidence of seromas or hematomas.[1,2]

Patients may undergo either a mini-facelift (short scar facelift) or a full lower facelift to address the neck. A mini-facelift for our patients does not involve direct submental work. Incisions are placed in front of the ear in a posttragal position, post-auricularly, and, if needed, across the auriculocephalic angle and back into the hairline for a limited extent. Undermining is carried out as a short flap of 5 to 6 cm. Superficial musculoaponeurotic system (SMAS) imbrication is performed. Flaps are then advanced posteriorly in front of the ear and superiorly behind and redundant skin is removed.

A full lower facelift involves direct submental work, typically platysma plication as well as submental liposuction. Incisions are longer, typically into the temporal hairline and posteriorly along the occipital hairline allowing for more skin redraping. Undermining is completed with a long flap that extends 7 to 8 cm anterior and posterior to the ear and is continuous with undermining submentally. An extended superficial musculoaponeurotic system (SMAS) imbrication is performed. Flaps are advanced as with a mini-facelift and redundant skin is removed.

Fibrin Sealant Procedure

Following the facelift procedure and prior to closure the ARTISS fibrin sealant is applied.

- The packaged syringe sprayer is stored in a freezer and must be thawed prior to use.

- The syringe unit containing the thrombin and fibrinogen chambers (**Fig. 2**) is attached to the Easy Spray Unit (**Fig. 3**), which provides controlled pressurized air.

- With the flaps elevated and retracted, ARTISS is sprayed over the raw dissected surfaces as a thin even layer. A distance of 10–15 cm is recommended, but closer application is possible at reduced pressure settings. Typically less than 1 mL per side is used.

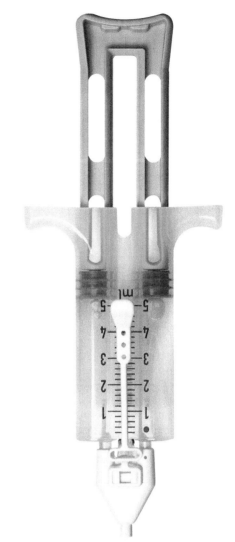

Fig. 2. Syringe sprayers. (*Courtesy of* Baxter Healthcare, Wayne, PA; with permission.)

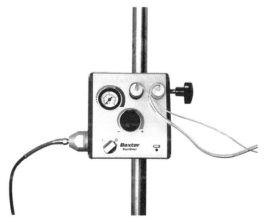

Fig. 3. Easy spray unit. (*Courtesy of* Baxter Healthcare, Wayne, PA; with permission.)

- The flaps are then immediately placed in position with staples at key points and pressure is applied

- Lap sponges are utilized to provide even pressure and prevent finger marks.

- Pressure is applied for 3 minutes after each application to both sides and submentally.

- Closure is performed after each application in a layered, plastics fashion.

- A light compression dressing is applied to finish the procedure.

Outcomes of Fibrin Sealant

Our own experience with ARTISS has mirrored others who have seen less bruising and swelling and a quicker recovery. We have had no hematomas or seromas in patients receiving the fibrin sealant. At the American Academy of Facial Plastic Surgery 2013 annual meeting, 2 reports, one by Farrior[12] with ARTISS and a second more long-term study with TISSEEL by Caniglia[13] found similar results. Most of our patients receiving ARTISS have been in the mini-facelift category (**Figs. 4** and **5**); however, we are using the fibrin sealant increasingly on patients with full lower facelift as well (**Fig. 6**). We believe that fibrin sealants are a beneficial addition to procedures involving rejuvenation of the neck.

CHIN AUGMENTATION

Although chin augmentation is commonly performed in conjunction with rhinoplasty, it, too, contributes to the contour of the neck. Microgenia, retrognathia, and resorption can create an obtuse cervicomental angle by decreasing the distance between the hyoid and chin.[14,15] Furthermore, a well-projected chin serves as a focal point for which the superficial musculoaponeurotic system (SMAS) may be suspended and the skin redraped during a rhytidectomy.[16] Therefore, it is important to recognize any deficiencies of the chin before a neck rejuvenation procedure. For women, the mentum should be 1 to 2 mm posterior to the plane of the lower lip vermilion border and, for men, it should be at or slightly in front of this plane.

There are a variety of techniques used in augmenting the chin. Augmentation with facial implants is popular among facial plastic surgeons. Implants are classified by the source from which they are derived. Autogenous grafts, such as bone and cartilage, are harvested from the patient.

Autogenous grafts, however, suffer from limited availability, donor site morbidity, and resorption over time. Homologous grafts, such as cadaveric rib, are harvested from cadavers and are then irradiated to remove pathogens. Homografts yield no donor site morbidity and are widely available, but are plagued by patient fear of disease transmission and also unpredictable resorption. Alloplastic implants are made from synthetic materials. Alloplastic grafts are widely available, avoid donor site morbidity, and do not transmit disease. The ideal alloplastic implant should be inert, noninflammatory, noncarcinogenic, nonallergenic, nonreactive material that is easily obtained, molded, implanted, secured, and removed if needed. The material should be pliable enough to conform to different shapes and resist distortion. It should not cause erosion of nearby structures.[17,18] A variety of materials are used for alloplastic mentoplasty.

Expanded Polytetrafluorethylene

Expanded polytetrafluoroethylene (ePTFE or Gore-Tex; W. L. Gore and Associates, Flagstaff, AZ) was the first biosynthetic material designed for implantation in humans. It is nondegradable, inert, pliable, and easily cut to shape. It has small pores, allowing for fibrovascular ingrowth and stability after placement. Godin and colleagues[19] reviewed 324 cases of ePTFE used in augmentation mentoplasty, and found an overall infection rate of 0.62% and no resorption. On the other hand, Shi and colleagues[20] reported a case of severe bone resorption underneath an ePTFE implant that they attributed to mentalis muscle hyperactivity. Others criticize that ePTFE is too soft and pliable.[21]

Porous Polyethylene

Porous polyethylene (Medpor; Stryker Corp, Kalamazoo, MI) is another commonly used material. It is nonallergenic, nonantigenic, nonabsorbable, highly stable, easy to fixate, and available in a variety of shapes and sizes. Its porous nature allows for fibrovascular ingrowth and stabilization of the graft. Porous polyethylene, however, suffers from poor pliability and therefore may not contour well to the mandible. Niechajev[22] reported no infections in 28 Medpor chin implants and only 3 infections overall using Medpor facial implants. Gui and colleagues[23] reported no infections or alloplastic reactions to the Medpor chin implants in 150 chin augmentation procedures.

Polyamide Mesh

Polyamide mesh (Supramid; Ethicon, Somerville, NJ) is an organopolymer related to nylon or

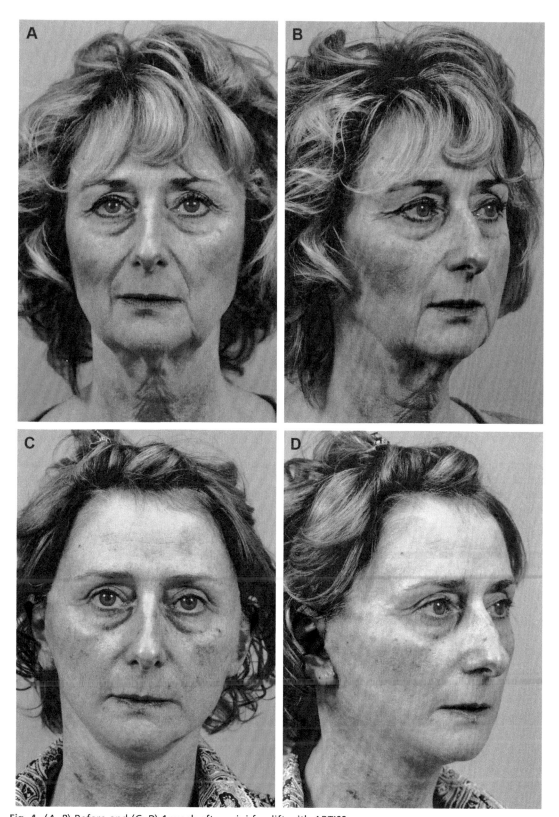

Fig. 4. (*A, B*) Before and (*C, D*) 1 week after mini-facelift with ARTISS.

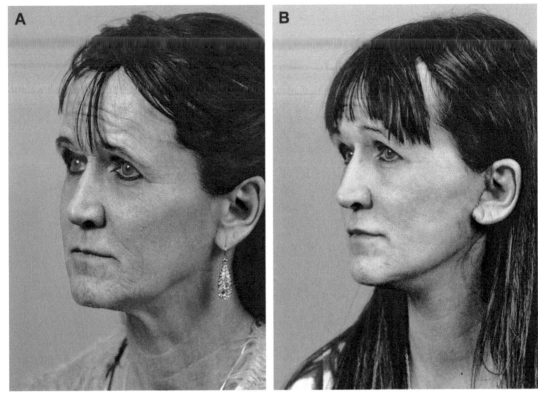

Fig. 5. (A) Before and (B) 1 week after mini-facelift with ARTISS.

polyester fiber. It is flexible, easily cut and shaped, and allows for fibrovascular ingrowth. Polyamide mesh, however, has been found to elicit an intense foreign body response resulting in chronic inflammation.[24] Beekhuis[25] reported generally favorable results in more than 200 patients using polyamide mesh for nasal and chin implants, but did note occasional loss of bulk due to resorption.

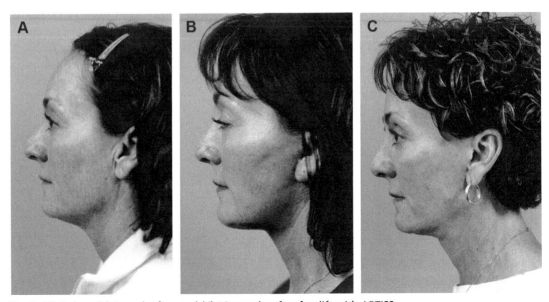

Fig. 6. (A) Before, (B) 1 week after, and (C) 10 months after facelift with ARTISS.

Silicone Rubber

Silicone rubber is a popular implant that is commonly used in various parts of the body. It is a nonporous material, therefore it does not allow for fibrovascular ingrowth. A local inflammatory response results in thin fibrous capsule formation around the implant itself. If the implant is mobile, then a seroma can form. If the tissue overlying the implant is thinned, then extrusion may occur. Various reports have found that bone resorption occurred underneath the implant over time.[26–28] Infection rates were low for both external and intraoral placement of the silicone implant.[27,29]

Mersilene Mesh

Mersilene mesh (polyamide nylon mesh or polyester fiber; Ethicon) was first introduced in 1950. It is composed of nonabsorbable nylon polyester fibers that are woven into multifilament strands of polyethylene terephthalate. The pore size of the mesh is large enough to allow tissue ingrowth, which helps to secure the implant. Mersilene mesh is inert, noninflammatory, noncarcinogenic, and nonreactive. It has great tensile strength to resist distortion, yet it is pliable enough to conform to the bony skeleton. In addition, it provides a natural appearance and is essentially nonpalpable.[18,21] Studies by McCollough and colleagues[30] and Gross and colleagues[21] showed that Mersilene is a safe, implantable material with low infection rates.

Our preferred material for chin augmentation is the Mersilene mesh. Here, we describe our approach and technique. The need for chin augmentation first starts with evaluation of the patient. The standard 3 views are obtained in the Frankfort horizontal plane with normal occlusion. Chin projection is evaluated by dropping a vertical line from the lower lip. The depth of the labiomental sulcus is also noted and should be approximately 4 mm posterior to this line. Cephalometric radiographs are generally not needed. Contraindications to augmentation include severe microgenia (requiring >10 mm of projection), shortened mandibular height with lower lip protrusion, severe periodontal disease, preexisting anatomic or functional impairment of the oral sphincter, age younger than 15 years, and prosthetic heart valves or ventriculoperitoneal shunts.[21]

Our technique for creation of the implant is well described elsewhere.[21,30] The Mersilene mesh is supplied in a single 30 × 30-cm sheet. A 5 × 2-cm template is placed onto the outstretched sheet and the mesh is folded onto itself 9 times to create a rectangular shape that is 10 layers thick. The template is then removed. To create a double implant, an additional step is required. A 5 × 1-cm template is used to create a smaller implant of the same shape and thickness (10 layers). The smaller implant is then sutured on top of the larger implant to create a double implant that is 20 sheets thick. A triple implant is created by adding an additional 5 × 2-cm implant. The implants are sutured together with a 5-0 polyglyconate suture in a running horizontal mattress fashion. The implants are then packaged, labeled, and steam sterilized before implantation.

The Mersilene implant can be placed via an intra-oral or submental approach. Prior to the incision, intravenous cefazolin is administered (for both approaches). In both techniques, the implant is placed between the pogonion and menton, which yields the most natural chin profile. We will first describe the intra-oral approach.

Implant Placement Via Intraoral Approach

Before the incision, intravenous cefazolin is administered (for both approaches).

- A 2.5 cm incision is made through the inner aspect of the lower lip at least 1 cm above and parallel to the gingival labial sulcus.

- A Freer elevator is used to bluntly dissect over the mandibular symphysis in a subperiosteal plane.

- Dissection is carried inferior towards the lower border of the mandible and lateral towards the mental foramen ensuring to stay inferior to the mental nerves.

- The appropriate sized implant is selected.

- The implant is then cut and trimmed to create a tapered lateral border.

- The implant is soaked in a solution of bacitracin (50,000 U) and gentamycin sulfate (80 mg).

- The soft tissue is retracted and the implant is placed into position under direct visualization.
- Inspection and palpation confirms the proper placement and final chin projection.

- The periosteum is closed such that it prevents implant migration.

- The incision is closed in layers with the surgeon's choice of suture technique and material.

Implant Placement Via Submental Approach

- For the submental approach, a 2 cm transverse incision is made just posterior to the submental crease.

- Sharp dissection is carried down to the periosteum of the mandibular symphysis.

- A subperiosteal plane is developed by blunt dissection centrally and laterally, ensuring to not injure the mental nerves.

- As with the intra-oral approach, the implant is shaped and placed under direct visualization and confirmed by manual palpation and inspection.

- The periosteum is closed to prevent migration of the implant.

- The skin is closed in layers.

Post Procedure

- After the incision is closed, Mastisol (Ferndale Laboratories; Ferndale, MI) and Micropore tan tape (3M Corp, Minneapolis, MN) is applied to the skin overlying the anterior aspect of the chin.

- A circumferential head dressing encompassing the chin is applied using 4×4 inch 6 ply Curity gauze sponges (Covidien, Mansfield, MA, USA) and 4 1/2 inches × 4 1/8 yards 6 ply Kerlix (Covidien, Mansfield, MA, USA) for mild compression and hemostasis.

- The dressing is removed the following day.

- For the intra-oral approach, the patient is instructed to rinse their mouth with hydrogen peroxide and water following each meal.

- All patients are prescribed 500 mg of oral cephalexin twice daily for 5 days.

- The patient follows up in 1 week, 1 month, 3 months, 6 months, and each year thereafter.

Outcomes of Surgical Approaches

While the approach is largely based on surgeon preference and comfort, there are potential benefits to each approach. The obvious benefit of an intraoral approach is the lack of an external scar. The malposition rate is lower with this approach due to improved exposure; however, the infection rate is slightly higher. Failure to reapproximate the mentalis muscle can lead to chin ptosis.[31]

Chin augmentation allows the achievement of a better neckline in patients with microgenia. Benefits can be seen with patients undergoing simply liposuction (Fig. 7), as well as those undergoing a full lower facelift (Fig. 8). Evaluation of chin projection and augmentation when indicated is a critical part of optimal neck rejuvenation.

SUBMANDIBULAR GLAND PTOSIS

A youthful and aesthetically pleasing neck requires a well-defined inferior border of the mandible. The inferior border of the mandible is lined by a shadow from the bony mentum to the mandibular angle. This line should be free of blunting from submandibular gland ptosis and uninterrupted by jowl overhang.[32] Specifically, aging can result in submandibular gland fullness and increased laxity of the neck fascial layers resulting in submandibular gland ptosis.[33] Although rhytidectomy and platysma plication can address the laxity issue, the results are not long lasting.[33,34] Furthermore, prominence of the gland can be unveiled after those procedures.[35] To address the ptotic submandibular gland, Guyuron and colleagues[34] proposed a basket submandibular gland suspension technique using deep temporal fascia to suspend the gland. Although their technique was effective at 1.8 years of follow-up, complications included infection, temporary lingual nerve paresthesia, and palpable suspension sutures. We also note that their technique does not address the hypertrophic gland.

For those with a hypertrophic gland, the best treatment is either partial or total resection of the gland.[33–35] This form of treatment, however, is met with great reluctance because of the proximity of the submandibular gland to important neurovascular structures (ie, marginal mandibular branch of the facial nerve, hypoglossal nerve, lingual nerve and artery, and facial artery and vein). Review of the recent literature demonstrated low rates of temporary and permanent nerve injury in patients undergoing excision for submandibular gland disease.[36–39] In patients who underwent partial submandibular gland excision for cosmetic reasons, there were no long-term complications.[34,35] Therefore, in the hands of a fully trained otolaryngologist, excision of the submandibular gland poses minimal risk to the patient.

Another factor to consider in planning for the removal of the submandibular gland is placement of the incision and the resultant scar. Although only 2.5% of patients in the general population

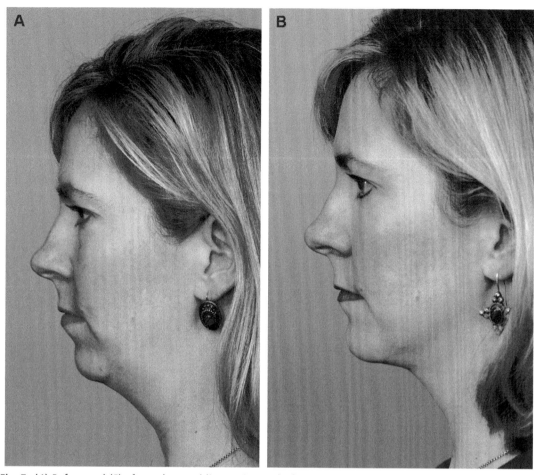

Fig. 7. (A) Before and (B) after submental liposuction with chin augmentation.

reported dissatisfaction with the final appearance of the scar via a standard transcervical approach,[38] that rate is likely to be much higher in the cosmetic patient. Other, less conspicuous, approaches include submental, retroauricular, transoral, endoscopic-assisted transoral, and endoscopic-assisted submental.[40]

Several investigators have described the intraoral dissection.[41,42] One of the biggest advantages of this technique is the avoidance of an external scar; however, an intraoral dissection does require more operative time initially and the resultant scar in the floor of mouth can cause asymmetric movement of the tongue. Roh[39] reported his experience with the retroauricular approach to the submandibular gland. Although the incision is longer, patients were ultimately more satisfied with the scar, operative times were not significantly longer, and complications were comparable with the traditional transcervical approach. Roh[43] also presented his experience with the submental approach compared with the traditional transcervical

approach. Although his study was small, the submental approach yielded similar operative times, similar incision length, low rates of complications, and improved patient satisfaction with the resultant scar. Singer and Sullivan[33] provide an excellent anatomic review and technique description of the submental approach.

Submandibular gland hypertrophy and ptosis create a challenge for the facial plastic surgeon. Although options exist for correction, they are associated with either significant risks or an additional surgical incision and resulting scar. We do not recommend submandibular gland modification as part of elective neck rejuvenation.

HYOID BONE POSITION

The position of the hyoid bone contributes greatly to the overall appearance and contour of one's neck.[14] A superior and posterior hyoid bone results in a more acute and attractive cervicomental angle, whereas an inferiorly and anteriorly

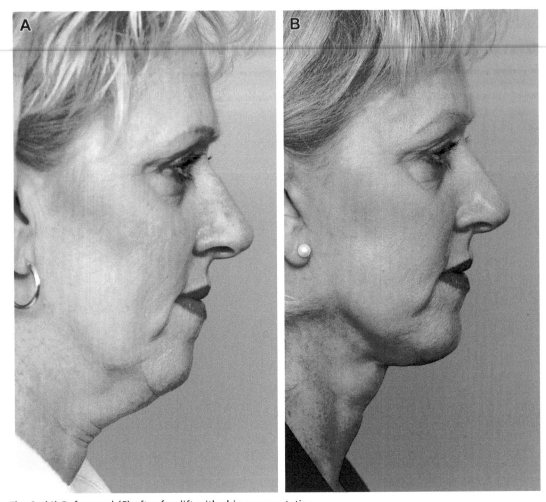

Fig. 8. (A) Before and (B) after facelift with chin augmentation.

positioned hyoid bone can create an obtuse cervi-comental angle.

Guyuron[14] reviewed images of 54 patients and concluded that a balanced neck is one in which the caudal border of the hyoid body is located at or above a line parallel to the Frankfort horizontal line passing through the pogonion. He also showed that by dividing the attachments of the anterior digastric, geniohyoid, and mylohyoid muscles from the mandibular symphysis allowed for posterior and superior relocation of the hyoid bone, resulting in a more aesthetically pleasing neck contour. Guyuron[14] also observed that lengthening the anterior-posterior distance of the hyoid bone to the chin would better define the cervicomental angle. Although not described in the current clinical literature, Knipper and col-leagues[44] conducted a cadaveric study in which they plicated the digastric tendon, which resulted

in a posterior-superior displacement of the hyoid bone. Their study resulted in a decrease of the cer-vicomental angle and also elevation of the hyoid bone.

Although we recognize the importance of hyoid position, we have no experience nor do we recom-mend modification procedures to the hyoid. Further studies may be warranted to investigate the clinical effectiveness of these procedures in patients who have a low and anteriorly positioned hyoid but desire a more aesthetically pleasing neckline.

SUMMARY

There are a myriad of techniques that can help to enhance the aesthetic result of neck rejuvenation procedures. Fibrin sealants, such as TISSEEL and ARTISS, can obviate the need for drains after rhytidectomy and thus improve the patient's experience. We believe their use also decreases postoperative swelling and bruising and decreases the incidence of seromas and hematomas. Although chin augmentation is a common adjunctive procedure in patients receiving rhinoplasty, it plays an equally important role in patients who desire a more youthful neckline and should not be overlooked. Despite improvements in rhytidectomy techniques and excellent long-term results, there exist areas of the neck that are difficult to treat. Hypertrophic submandibular glands and malposition of the hyoid bone continue to create challenges for the facial plastic surgeon. We look forward to future research and improvements in surgical technique to further enhance neck rejuvenation in our patients.

REFERENCES

1. Hester TR, Gerut ZE, Shire JR, et al. Exploratory, randomized, controlled, phase 2 study to evaluate the safety and efficacy of adjuvant fibrin sealant VH S/D 4 S-Apr (ARTISS) in patients undergoing rhytidectomy. Aesthet Surg J 2013; 33(3):323–33.

2. Hester TR, Shire JR, Nguyen DB, et al. Randomized, controlled, phase 3 study to evaluate the safety and efficacy of fibrin sealant VH S/D 4 s-apr (Artiss) to improve tissue adherence in subjects undergoing rhytidectomy. Aesthet Surg J 2013;33(4):487–96.

3. Gosain AK, Lyon VB, Plastic Surgery Educational Foundation DATA Committee. The current status of tissue glues: part II. For adhesion of soft tissues. Plast Reconstr Surg 2002;110(6):1581–4.

4. Ellis DA, Pelausa EO. Fibrin glue in facial plastic and reconstructive surgery. J Otolaryngol 1988;17(2): 74–7.

5. Oliver DW, Hamilton 3A, Figle AA, et al. A prospective, randomized, double-blind trial of the use of fibrin sealant for face lifts. Plast Reconstr Surg 2001;108(7):2101–5 [discussion: 2106–7].

6. Kamer FM, Nguyen DB. Experience with fibrin glue in rhytidectomy. Plast Reconstr Surg 2007;120(4): 1045–51 [discussion: 1052].

7. Zoumalan D, Rizk CC. Hematoma rates in drainless deep-plane face-lift surgery with and without the use of fibrin glue. Arch Facial Plast Surg 2008; 10(2):103–7.

8. Fezza JP, Cartwright M, Mack W, et al. The use of aerosolized fibrin glue in face-lift surgery. Plast Reconstr Surg 2002;110(2):658–64 [discussion: 665–6].

9. Powell DM, Chang E, Farrior EH. Recovery from deep-plane rhytidectomy following unilateral wound treatment with autologous platelet gel: a pilot study. Arch Facial Plast Surg 2001;3(4):245–50.

10. Marchac D, Sandor G. Face lifts and sprayed fibrin glue: an outcome analysis of 200 patients. Br J Plast Surg 1994;47(5):306–9.

11. Marchac D, Greensmith AL. Early postoperative efficacy of fibrin glue in face lifts: a prospective randomized trial. Plast Reconstr Surg 2005;115(3): 911–6 [discussion: 917–8].

12. Farrior E. Long term Use of Fibrin Sealants in Rhytidectomy. Presented at AAFPRS Fall meeting. New Orleans, October 19–21, 2013.

13. Polle and Caniglia. Evaluation of Fibrin Sealants and Postoperative Hematoma/Seroma Rates in Rhtidectomy. Presented at AAFPRS Fall meeting. New Orleans, October 20, 2013.

14. Guyuron B. Problem neck, hyoid bone, and submental myotomy. Plast Reconstr Surg 1992;90(5): 830–7 [discussion: 838–40].

15. Mendelson B, Wong CH. Changes in the facial skeleton with aging: implications and clinical applications in facial rejuvenation. Aesthetic Plast Surg 2012;36(4):753–60.

16. Konuk O, Kurtulmusoglu M, Knatova Z, et al. Unsuccessful lacrimal surgery: causative factors and results of surgical management in a tertiary referral center. Ophthalmologica 2010;224:361–6.

17. Romo T 3rd, Lanson BG. Chin augmentation. Facial Plast Surg Clin North Am 2008;16(1):69–77, vi.

18. Zeph RD. Custom-designed chin augmentation. Facial Plast Surg Clin North Am 2008;16(1):79–85, vi.

19. Godin M, Costa L, Romo T, et al. Gore-Tex chin implants: a review of 324 cases. Arch Facial Plast Surg 2003;5(3):224–7.

20. Shi L, Zhang ZY, Tang XJ. Severe bone resorption in expanded polytetrafluoroethylene chin augmentation. J Craniofac Surg 2013;24(5):1711–2.

21. Gross EJ, Hamilton MM, Ackermann K, et al. Mersilene mesh chin augmentation. A 14-year experience. Arch Facial Plast Surg 1999;1(3):183–9 [discussion: 190].

22. Niechajev I. Facial reconstruction using porous high-density polyethylene (Medpor): long-term results. Aesthetic Plast Surg 2012;36(4):917–27.

23. Gui L, Huang L, Zhang Z. Genioplasty and chin augmentation with Medpore implants: a report of 650 cases. Aesthetic Plast Surg 2008;32(2): 220–6.

24. Quatela VC, Chow J. Synthetic facial implants. Facial Plast Surg Clin North Am 2008;16(1):1–10, v.

25. Beekhuis GJ. Augmentation mentoplasty with polyamide mesh. Update. Arch Otolaryngol 1984; 110(6):364–7.

26. Saleh HA, Lohuis PJ, Vuyk HD. Bone resorption after alloplastic augmentation of the mandible. Clin Otolaryngol Allied Sci 2002;27(2):129–32.

27. Vuyk HD. Augmentation mentoplasty with solid silicone. Clin Otolaryngol Allied Sci 1996;21(2): 106–18.

28. Pearson DC, Sherris DA. Resorption beneath silastic mandibular implants. Effects of placement and pressure. Arch Facial Plast Surg 1999;1(4):261–4 [discussion: 265].

20. Aynehchi BB, Burstein DH, Parhiscar A, et al. Vertical incision intraoral silicone chin augmentation. Otolaryngol Head Neck Surg 2012;146(1):553 0.

30. McCollough EG, Hom DB, Weigel MT, et al. Augmentation mentoplasty using Mersilene mesh. Arch Otolaryngol Head Neck Surg 1990;116(10): 1154–8.

31. Cuzalina LA, Hlavacek MR. Complications of facial implants. Oral Maxillofac Surg Clin North Am 2009; 21(1):91–104, vi–vii.

32. Ellenbogen R, Karlin JV. Visual criteria for success in restoring the youthful neck. Plast Reconstr Surg 1980;66(6):826–37.

33. Singer DP, Sullivan PK. Submandibular gland I: an anatomic evaluation and surgical approach to submandibular gland resection for facial rejuvenation. Plast Reconstr Surg 2003;112(4):1150–4 [discussion: 1155–6].

34. Guyuron B, Jackowe D, Iamphongsai S. Basket submandibular gland suspension. Plast Reconstr Surg 2008;122(3):938–43.

35. de Pina DP, Quinta WC. Aesthetic resection of the submandibular salivary gland. Plast Reconstr Surg 1991;88(5):779–87 [discussion: 788].

36. Preuss SF, Klussmann JP, Wittekindt C, et al. Submandibular gland excision: 15 years of experience. J Oral Maxillofac Surg 2007;65(5): 953–7.

37. Hernando M, Echarri RM, Taha M, et al. Surgical complications of submandibular gland excision. Acta Otorrinolaringol Esp 2012;63(1):42–6.

38. Springborg LK, Moller MN. Submandibular gland excision: long term clinical outcome in 130 patients operated in a single institution. Eur Arch Otorhinolaryngol 2013;270(4):1441–6.

39. Roh JL. Removal of the submandibular gland by a retroauricular approach. Arch Otolaryngol Head Neck Surg 2006;132(7):783–7.

40. Beahm DD, Peleaz L, Nuss DW, et al. Surgical approaches to the submandibular gland: a review of literature. Int J Surg 2009;7(6):503–9.

41. Hong KH, Kim YK. Intraoral removal of the submandibular gland: a new surgical approach. Otolaryngol Head Neck Surg 2000;122(6):798–802.

42. Smith AD, Elahi MM, Kawamoto HK Jr, et al. Excision of the submandibular gland by an intraoral approach. Plast Reconstr Surg 2000;105(6):2092–5.

43. Roh JL. Removal of the submandibular gland by a submental approach: a prospective, randomized, controlled study. Oral Oncol 2008;44(3): 295–300.

44. Knipper P, Mitz V, Lemerle JP. Experimental cervicoplasty: correction of the cervicomental angle by postero-superior suspension of the hyoid bone. A study of 20 anatomical dissections. Ann Chir Plast Esthet 1996;41(1):37–44 [in French].

Techniques for Rejuvenation of the Neck Platysma

Edward Farrior, MD[a],*, Lindsay Eisler, MD[b],
Harry V. Wright, MD, MS[a]

KEYWORDS

- Neck • Neck lift • Facial rejuvenation • Cervicomental angle • Rhytidectomy • Platysmaplasty
- Submental liposuction

KEY POINTS

- It is imperative to identify the goals of the patient and his or her desired outcome.
- Careful examination of the patient is important to determine if correction can meet the patient's goals.
- Surgical correction is focused on re-establishing the cervicomental angle, decreasing submental fullness, eliminating jowls, and platysmal banding.
- There are multiple adjuvant procedures that can be employed to augment surgical correction.
- Surgical correction is not without risks, and complications include hematoma, nerve injury, flap necrosis, and scar irregularities.

INTRODUCTION

Aesthetic rejuvenation of the neck focuses on restoring the shape and contour of the neck, with special attention to redefining the cervicomental angle. As individuals age, the neck skin loses elasticity; submental fat becomes abundant and ptotic, and the platysmal muscle adherence to the subplatysmal fat and tongue musculature weakens. Additionally, muscle tone atrophies, and the submandibular glands descend. As a result, the cervicomental angle becomes blunted; the angle and inferior border of the mandible lose definition, and there is an abundance of skin in the submentum. These changes embody individuals' dissatisfaction with the appearance of their neck and their desire to seek surgical correction. Various surgical and nonsurgical techniques are used alone or in combination to address the aging process of the neck and deliver the desired result of restoration.

TREATMENT GOALS AND PLANNED OUTCOME

The primary goal of surgery is to restore the youthful appearance of the neck. This includes re-establishing a refined cervicomental angle, decreasing adiposity and fullness in the submentum, obliterating platysmal banding, eliminating jowling, and recreating definition of the mandible. Multiple studies have defined the appearance of a youthful neck. Some of the characteristics include an acute cervicomental angle between 105° and 120°, a distinct inferior border of the mandible, visible anterior borders of the sternocleidomastoid muscles, and a noticeable thyroid cartilage and subthyroid depression.[1,2]

Baker has developed a classification system of the aging process in the neck and lower face.[3] This organizes patients into 4 subtypes based on the severity of the jowl and neck. Type 1 patients have slight cervical skin laxity with submental fat

[a] Department of Otolaryngology-Head and Neck Surgery, University of South Florida, 12901 Bruce B. Downs Boulevard, MDC 73, Tampa, FL 33612, USA; [b] Department of Otolaryngology-Head and Neck Surgery, Geisinger Medical Center, 100 North Academy Avenue, Danville, PA 17822, USA
* Corresponding author. 2908 West Azeele Street, Tampa, FL 33609–3110.
E-mail address: ed@drfarrior.com

Facial Plast Surg Clin N Am 22 (2014) 243–252
http://dx.doi.org/10.1016/j.fsc.2014.01.012
1064-7406/14/$ – see front matter © 2014 Elsevier Inc. All rights reserved.

and early jowls. Type 2 patients have moderate cervical skin laxity, moderate jowl, and submental fat. Type 3 patients have moderate cervical skin laxity, but with significant jowling and active platysmal banding. Type 4 patients have loose, redundant cervical skin and folds below the cricoid, significant jowls, and active platysmal bands.

Classification systems as the one described can categorize patients and help to highlight the key anatomic findings of different patients and their primary need for rejuvenation. It is important to distinguish the need for correction so that the correct method of neck rejuvenation can be used to target the specific anatomic finding. There are many methods that have been described for neck rejuvenation. Many of these are variants on larger themes and include both surgical and nonsurgical options. These range from chemodenervation, laser skin resurfacing, submental liposuction, skin tightening procedures, skin excision procedures, platysmaplasty, suspension sutures, and digastric modification. It is important to identify the need for correction as well as the patient's goals of surgery to determine the best course of rejuvenation.

Ideal candidates for surgery are patients with strong bone structure with a normal position of the hyoid bone and good chin projection, as well as skin of medium thickness that has maintained its elasticity. Certain anatomic considerations can alter the potential outcome. Obtaining a sharp cervicomental angle can be hampered in patients with low positioned hyoid bones as well as retrognathic patients. There is little that can be done in the patient with a low positioned hyoid bone, but in the retrognathic patient, augmentation mentoplasty should be considered. Neck definition can also be suboptimal in patients with thick skin or excessive subcutaneous adiposity.

This article addresses cervical rhytidectomy as well as adjuvant techniques that can be employed to reach the desired goal of the patient and surgeon.

PREOPERATIVE PLANNING AND PREPARATION

Prior to consultation, the patient is asked to fill out a detailed questionnaire. Routine historical questions are asked to obtain information about their medical, surgical, social, and family history. On the day of the initial consultation, patients are photographed for documentation and to aid in preoperative planning. The standard photographic views include full-face frontal view, right and left oblique views, and right and left lateral views. All photographs are taken in the Frankfurt horizontal line using a single lens reflex (SLR) with appropriate medium blue background and balanced cross-lighting

It is imperative to determine the patient's goal and desire for correction and to define which modality of correction will target and correct his or her desire for rejuvenation. For instance, if a patient's primary concern is an abundance of submental adiposity and mild jowling, but the patient has maintained skin elasticity, submental lipectomy would be a reasonable approach versus cervical rhytidectomy. However, for patients with blunting of anatomic landmarks and redundant ptotic cervical skin, a cervical rhytidectomy is the most reasonable approach.

A complete medical history should be obtained. Patients with a history cardiovascular disease are not precluded from surgery but require preoperative clearance by their cardiologist. Also, the overall health and ability of the patient to tolerate anesthetic and surgical intervention should be assessed. All patients are given an American Society of Anesthesiologists (ASA) classification. There are not many systemic diseases that proscribe patients from cervical rhytidectomy. Relative contraindications to surgery include advanced autoimmune diseases relating to the skin of the face, a history of systemic isotretinoin use, and medications or true allergy that would impact the ability to use local anesthetic. Obesity is not a contraindication to surgical correction; however, if a significant weight loss is planned in the near future, it is advised that surgery is postponed until after the patient's desired weight has been achieved. A history of full-course radiation treatment to neck and preauricular area is an absolute contraindication to cervical rhytidectomy. The physical examination should be focused on the neck and jaw line. The quality of the skin is assessed, including thickness, degree of elasticity, and severity of dermatochalasis. Skin laxity in the jowl, submental, and cervicomental angle is also evaluated. The position of the hyoid bone and chin position is noted. Identifying these key findings allows the surgeon the opportunity to discuss potential limitations of surgical correction and ensures the patient has reasonable postoperative expectations.

All of the patient's questions should be answered. The procedure should be outlined in detail, including incision placement. The risks, benefits, potential complications, alternatives and limitations must be comprehensively discussed prior to conclusion of the consultation. All patients undergoing surgery should be asked to suspend all anticoagulants and vitamin supplements that may cause clotting abnormalities prior to surgery.

PATIENT POSITIONING

On the day of surgery, the planned incision lines are marked with patient in the upright and seated position. The incision is placed in a trichophytic fashion at the temporal and postauricular hairline. This location is chosen to avoid elevating the hairline following redraping of the skin. The senior author (EHF) does not change the position of the incision in male patients. The submental incision is marked as well and is always posterior to the natural chin crease to decrease visibility postoperatively.

The patient is placed supine on the operating table. Although patients are given the option of anesthesia, most patients choose a general anesthesia. Following intubation, 2 to 3 mm of hair is trimmed along the planned incision lines. The hair is then sectioned and secured with rubber bands around the planned incisions.

PROCEDURAL APPROACH
Neck Lift Procedure

A modified tumescent solution is prepared of 0.1% lidocaine with 1:1,000,000 epinephrine. The neck skin is infiltrated with 70 to 80 mL prior to beginning the procedure.

The procedure begins with a submental incision approximately 3 cm in length placed posterior to the natural submental crease. Placement of the incision here prevents scar contraction and unsightly postoperative deformity. A skin flap is elevated in the subcutaneous plane, extending inferiorly below the thyroid notch and laterally to the submandibular glands.

If the patient has excessive submental fat, this should be directly excised or aspirated. Subplatysmal fat should not be removed to prevent postoperative platysmal banding. A decision should then be made regarding need for platysmaplasty. Indications for platysmaplasty include severe preoperative platysmal banding and cobra neck deformity. If indicated, the plastysma muscle is elevated from the underlying tissue inferiorly to the hyoid bone. The platysma muscle is divided at the level of the hyoid bone or desired position of the cervicomental angle to recreate that angle. Historically, the senior author (EHF) has performed midline platysmal imbrication at this point; however, more recently, this has been abandoned to favor superolateral (rather than medial) vectors of motion. Hemostasis is then obtained with electrocautery. Once hemostasis has been achieved, the submental incision is closed with deep buried interrupted sutures.

Attention is then paid to the right side of the face. An additional 70 to 80 mL of 0.1% lidocaine with 1:1,000,000 epinephrine is infiltrated into the subcutaneous plane of the right-sided neck lift flap and incision. The postauricular incision is made, and skin flap elevation is performed sharply. The skin flap is elevated anteriorly using blunt dissection with scissors. A temporal trichophytic and tragal preauricular incision is then made, and the short skin flap is elevated anteriorly. A preauricular strip of areolar tissue and fat is trimmed from the zygomatic arch superiorly to approximately 2 cm below the angle of the mandible to delineate the posterior extent of the superficial musculoaponeurotic system (SMAS) flap. The superior extent of the SMAS flap is made by drawing the scalpel laterally from the inferior orbital rim to the tragal cartilage (**Fig. 1**). The deep plane is then elevated deep to the platysma muscle but superficial to the masseteric fascia (**Fig. 2**). The marginal mandibular branch of the facial nerve is identified

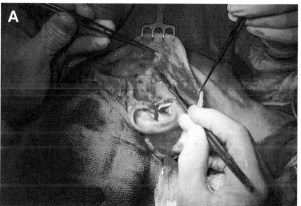
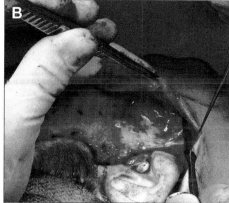

Fig. 1. Cervical rhytidectomy. (*A*) The superior extent of the SMAS flap is made by drawing the scalpel lightly across aponeurosis from the inferior orbital rim laterally to the tragal cartilage. (*B*) Note that the incision is placed in a trichophytic fashion at the temporal hairline to avoid elevation of the hairline.

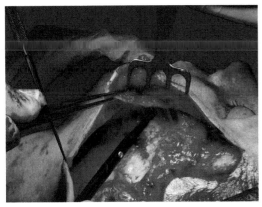

Fig. 2. Deep plane elevation is deep to platysma and superficial to the masseteric fascia.

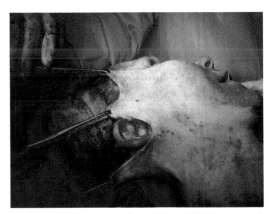

Fig. 3. Following suspension of the SMAS flap the skin flap is then redraped and marked, and redundant skin excised.

and protected during the dissection. The deep plane is suspended to the root of the lateral orbital rim, zygomatic arch, the mastoid cortex, fascia of the sternocleidomastoid, and preauricular soft tissue with a combination of permanent and slow-absorbing sutures. Hemostasis is achieved with electrocautery. The skin flap is then redraped (**Fig. 3**), marked, and all redundant skin excised. The skin flap is closed in layers with multiple deep buried interrupted sutures, and the epidermis is reapproximated with a fast-absorbing suture. An identical procedure is performed on the contralateral side. At the conclusion of the procedure, a pressure dressing is applied prior to extubation.

Direct Excision (Grecian Urn)

No approach to the cervicomental angle is more reproducible or consistently successful than the direct excision technique. Multiple pathologies

that contribute to the submental wattle, including excess skin and platysmal banding (**Fig. 4**A) and submental adiposity and skin excess (see **Fig. 4**B) can be addressed with direct excision. The Grecian Urn has been the senior author's (EHF) chosen approach to direct excision of submental soft tissue excess for over 25 years.

The patient is marked in the upright position. The amount of skin to be excised is marked conservatively, and, importantly, without stretching or recruiting additional skin to the midline. The transverse portions of the incision in the submental crease, at the desired cervicomental angle, and at the inferior extent of the wattle, are marked first (**Fig. 5**A). The skin is then pinched at the desired level of the cervicomental angle and marked (see **Fig. 5**B, green lines). This defines the width of the urn. Again, it is important to avoid recruiting additional lateral skin. These markings are position dependent; the remaining markings

A

B

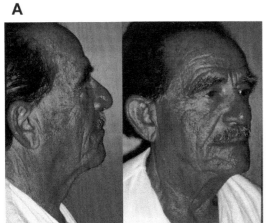
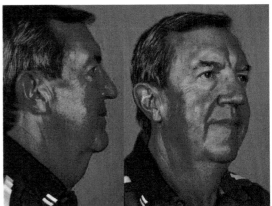

Fig. 4. Multiple pathologies can contribute to the submental wattle, all of which can be addressed with direct excision techniques. (*A*) Excess skin and platysmal banding. (*B*) Submental adiposity and excess skin.

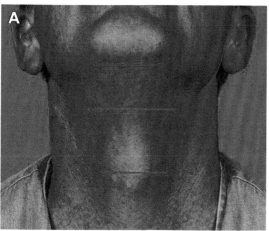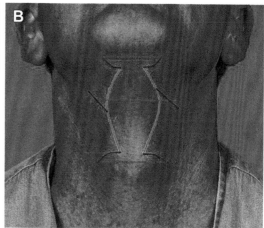

Fig. 5. Presurgical marking is performed with the patient in the upright position. (*A*) The transverse portion of the incision in the submental crease, at the desired cervicomental angle, and the inferior extent of the wattle are marked first. (*B*) The skin is pinched at the desired level of the cervicomental angle and marked to design the urn (*green lines*). The cervicomental angle-defining Z-plasty has limbs (*blue lines*) at least 2 cm long, 60° to vertical, and centered on the transverse line at the cervicomental angle with the flap limbs starting 1 cm both above and below the transverse.

can be performed with the patent supine prior to infiltration.

The cervicomental angle-defining Z-plasty is designed to have limbs that are at least 2 cm in length and 60° to vertical (see **Fig. 5**B, blue lines). The Z-plasty is centered on the transverse line at the cervicomental angle, with the flap limbs starting 1 cm above or 1 cm below the transverse. This assures symmetry and alignment. The proximal transverse segments of the superior and inferior extent of the vertical are designed to intersect the vertical excision with a length equal to half the length of the distal segment so that there are no length discrepancies, thereby avoiding a standing cutaneous cone.

After vasoconstriction has been obtained, the incisions are made using a #15 blade scalpel. All incisions on the border of the tissue to be excised are beveled away from the excision to create eversion at the time of closure. Once the incisions are made extending through the dermis and into the shallow subcuticular fat, the excess skin is resected in the subcutaneous plane just deep to the hair follicles (**Fig. 6**). The incisions for the limbs of the Z-plasty are then made perpendicular to the skin. Wide subcutaneous undermining is performed. The central fat is then grasped at the inferior extent of the desired excision. Direct fat excision is then performed using the Metzenbaum scissors. This will typically expose the anterior borders of the platysma muscle. If lateral fat excision is to be performed with liposuction, it can be performed through a submental stab incision prior to the excisional incisions being made or using an open technique after flap elevation.

Subplatysmal elevation is then performed bluntly with scissors. Bipolar electrocautery is used to cauterize the platysma laterally for 2 to 3 cm at the level of the transverse incision in the

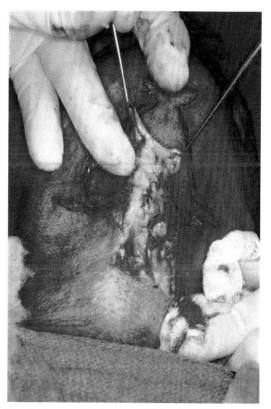

Fig. 6. Excess skin is resected in the subcutaneous plane just deep to the hair follicles.

platysma at the desired cervicomental angle (**Fig. 7**A). A midline imbrication of the platysma muscle is then performed in a vest-over-pants fashion using a 4–0 Maxon suture (see **Fig. 7**B).

The limbs of the Z-plasty are then transposed and secured with a Gillies corner stitch using 4–0 nylon. This helps to release tension for the rest of the closure. The central segment of the transverse incisions is also approximated with corner stitches. The subcutaneous closure is then performed with interrupted 4–0 and 5–0 Maxon. The epidermis is then approximated with 5–0 nylon in a running locking fashion (**Fig. 8**). The incision is further supported with suture strips and a supportive dressing (**Fig. 9**). The dressing remains in place for 24 to 48 hours and is then removed, leaving the suture strips in place for 5 to 7 days. The cutaneous sutures are removed at 5 to 7 days and are replaced with suture strips for an additional 5 to 7 days. In men, shaving is best initiated with an electric razor until irregularities in the wound margin have smoothed.

Cervical dermatochalasis, platysmal banding, and submental adiposity (**Figs. 10**A and **11**A) are effectively managed via Grecian Urn direct excision (see **Figs. 10**B and **11**B).

ADJUVANT TECHNIQUES FOR NECK REJUVENATION

Neuromodulators

Chemodenervation (botulinum toxin A) can be used in the platysma muscle to decrease platysmal banding. This can be used in combination with cervical rhytidectomy or as a stand-alone procedure for patients desiring a nonsurgical option. This would typically be recommended for patients without significant blunting of the cervicomental angle or significant jowling.

Laser Skin Resurfacing

The authors' preferred modality of skin resurfacing is the fractionated CO_2 laser. Both deep fractionated and skin resurfacing modalities are utilized. The entire anterior neck is resurfaced with overlapping in the vertical and horizontal plane. Because of the number of pilosebaceous units in the neck, the intensity of the laser is reduced compared with the fluence used for facial skin rejuvenation. Laser skin resurfacing is performed in combination with cervical rhytidectomy or submental liposuction and is typically performed concurrently. Laser skin resurfacing can also be used as a sole method

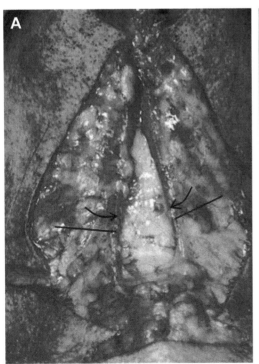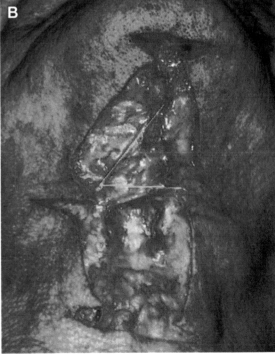

Fig. 7. The anterior borders of the platysma are exposed. Subplatysmal elevation is then performed bluntly with scissors. (*A*) Division of the platysma laterally for 2 to 3 cm occurs at the level of the transverse incision (the desired cervicomental angle) (*blue lines*). *Arrows* indicate the motion of the divided platysma for subsequent imbrication. (*B*) Midline imbrication of platysma is performed in a vest-over-pants fashion using a 4–0 Maxon suture.

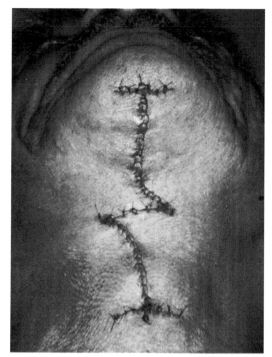

Fig. 8. The epidermis is approximated with 5–0 nylon running locking suture, which is removed at 5 to 7 days and replaced with suture strips for an additional 5 to 7 days.

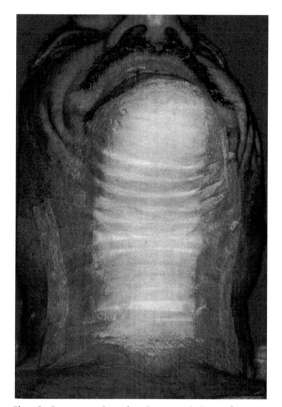

Fig. 9. Postoperative dressing consisting of suture strips and a supportive dressing (not shown). The dressing remains in place for 24 to 48 hours, the suture strips for 5 to 7 days.

for neck rejuvenation focused mainly on dermatochalasis and without excessive cervical skin, lipodystrophy, or platysmal banding.

Submental Liposuction

Submental liposuction is typically implemented for patients with excessive subcutaneous adipose tissue. The best results are in patients who have maintained good skin elasticity. This is performed with a blunt liposuction cannula through both a submental incision as well postauricular stab incisions. Blind passes are made prior to performing

A **B**

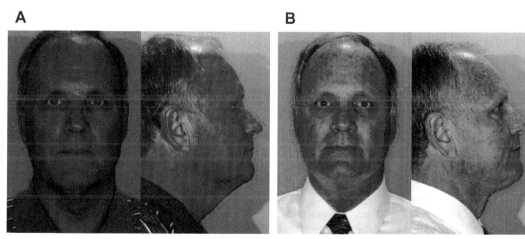

Fig. 10. Cervical dermatochalasis and platysmal banding in a patient before (A) and after (B) Grecian Urn direct excision.

A   **B**

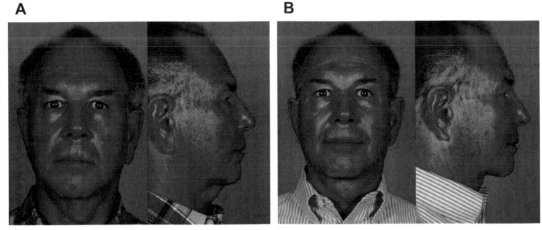

Fig. 11. Cervical dermatochalasis, platysmal banding, and submental adiposity in a patient before (*A*) and after (*B*) Grecian Urn direct excision.

liposuction. Care is taken to ensure the cannula faces toward the subcutaneous fat to prevent injury to the dermis, which can result in dimpling or tethering of the cervical skin after the procedure.

POTENTIAL COMPLICATIONS AND MANAGEMENT
Hematoma

The most common complication following cervical rhytidectomy is hematoma formation. The incidence varies and is reported to occur in 2% to 15% of patients.[4] The onset is typically characterized by pain and increasing facial edema. Risk factors for hematoma formation include hypertension, use of anticoagulant medication, vitamin E, and various herbal medications. Additionally, men and patients with Ehlers-Danlos syndrome are at higher risk.[5] The authors recommend halting all anticoagulant medication and herbal remedies 3 weeks prior to and following cervical rhytidectomy. Minor hematomas can frequently be managed conservatively with sterile needle aspiration followed by temporary pressure dressing once the collection has liquefied. Major or expanding hematomas typically occur in the first 12 hours postoperatively. These are heralded as true emergencies and typically require return to the operating room for surgical evacuation, control of hemostasis, drain placement, and postoperative pressure dressing placement. Skin flap necrosis can result with any significant delay in treatment. Unrecognized hematomas can ultimately lead to fibrosis underneath the skin flap causing puckering of the skin as well as discoloration. This can be treated with serial triamcinolone acetonide 10 mg/mL.

Flap Necrosis

Another potential complication of cervical rhytidectomy is skin flap necrosis. This can occur if the blood supply is compromised to the distal portion of the skin flap. Increased risk of skin flap necrosis is incurred by smoking, extended subcutaneous skin flap elevation, excessive tension, hematoma formation, and medical conditions such as peripheral vascular disease that predispose patients to vascular compromise.[6]

Nerve Injury

The most common nerve injured in a cervical rhytidectomy is the great auricular nerve. The incidence in the literature ranges from 1% to 7%.[7] If the injury goes unrepaired, the patient will suffer with regional hypoesthesia. The facial nerve is also at risk during cervical rhytidectomy. The most common branch affected is the marginal mandibular nerve. Facial nerve injury incidence for rhytidectomies ranges from 0.53% to 2.6% of patients per review of the literature.[4,8] Injury can be avoided by staying in the immediate subplatysmal plane and utilizing blunt dissection. Injury to the marginal mandibular nerve leads to permanent paresis of the depressor labii inferioris, resulting in an asymmetric smile.

Incision Irregularities

Loss of the temporal tuft of hair, alopecia, excessive dog-ear deformity, and a stair-stepping pattern of the hairline are all potential incision irregularities that can result from incision lines from a cervical rhytidectomy. The loss of the temporal tuft is avoided by placing the incision at the hairline. For patients with significant cervical skin redundancy, the incision is carried posteriorly along the hairline to alleviate a possible stair-stepping pattern. Alopecia is typically temporary and usually secondary to telogen effluvium. Potential solutions include scar revision and hair transplantation after allowing for enough time for scar maturation and potential regrowth of hair.

Earlobe Deformities

If the earlobe is not resuspended properly or there is undue tension on the skin flap, it can descend inferiorly while healing to form a Satyr's ear. This deformity is a telltale sign of rhytidectomy surgery. The best method for repair of the deformity is a V-Y scar revision. Revision should be delayed at least 6 months following rhytidectomy.

POSTPROCEDURAL CARE

Following the procedure, the patient must meet routine parameters prior to discharge. If the patient undergoes multiple combined procedures, overnight observation is recommended. The patient should be seen on postoperative day 1, and the pressure dressing should be removed. The incisions are cleaned with hydrogen peroxide, and triple antibiotic ointment is applied. The patient is counseled about wound care and cautioned about warning signs of potential complications. The patient is then seen weekly following the procedure until 1 month has passed. The patient is then seen at 3, 6, and 12 months after the procedure.

REHABILITATION AND RECOVERY

The authors recommend abstaining from rigorous physical activity for 3 weeks after the procedure. Vitamin supplements and medications that affect hemostasis should be withheld during this time period. It is also preferable if patients avoid strength training and direct, prolonged sun exposure for a total of 6 weeks.

OUTCOMES/CLINICAL RESULTS IN LITERATURE

Direct excision techniques for managing the neck in cosmetic facial rejuvenation offer an alternative or adjunct to face-lifting, liposuction, and platysmal imbrication. Importantly, they can create a defined cervicomental angle that is difficult to obtain with any other technique.

Proper patient selection and education are imperative as with all procedures to improve the neck. All of the approaches summarized in **Table 1** allow excellent access to the structures deep to the skin and therefore may incorporate various treatment options for the underlying platysma, fat (via direct excision or liposuction), and skeleton. A thorough summary has been published by Bitner and colleagues.[9]

Table 1
Direct excision techniques for addressing the cervicomental angle

Technique	Benefits	Drawbacks	Ref.
Linear excision	Simple, fast	Risk of leaving excess skin in the lateral direction and skin deficiency in the vertical direction, resulting in contraction bands with healing	10,11,12*
Z-plasty	E-K score for the cervicomental angle showed mean improvement from 0.6 to 3.3 points out of 5	3/17 (18%) patients underwent steroid injections for scar hypertrophy	13*
T-Z plasty	No particular benefits noted	Closure recommended to be "quite snug" otherwise insufficient tissue excised. Not recommended for routine use in women	14,15
Running W-plasty	Breaks up the vertically oriented portion of the scar	None noted	16*
Grecian Urn	No complications or revisions have been required	Technically complex direct technique	9*,17*

Abbreviation: E-K, Ellenbogen-Karlin.
* Indicates studies where the author(s) report no complications and no need for revision surgery.
Data from Refs.[9–17]

Direct excision techniques do not improve the jawline, however, and may worsen the appearance of an undulating jawline by creating a regional disharmony between the rejuvenated neck and the face.

SUMMARY

Neck rejuvenation is targeted at re-establishing the youthful contour of the neck. Focus is placed on defining the cervicomental angle, removing unwanted adipose tissue, excising excessive cervical skin, and eliminating platysmal banding. The authors have found that the most effective way to accomplish these goals is through a deep plane cervical rhytidectomy. Additional interventions can enhance the results of rhytidectomy or be utilized in patients desiring a nonsurgical option for rejuvenation. Careful consideration of the patient's anatomy and desired goal will dictate the correct course for rejuvenation.

REFERENCES

1. Ellenbogen R, Karlin JV. Visual criteria for success in restoring the youthful neck. Plast Reconstr Surg 1980;66(6):826–37.
2. Ramirez OM. Advanced considerations determining procedure selection in cervicoplasty. Part one: anatomy and aesthetics. Clin Plast Surg 2008;35(4):679–90.
3. Baker DC. Lateral SMASectomy, plication and short scar facelifts: indications and techniques. Clin Plast Surg 2008;35(4):533–50.
4. Rees A. Complications of rhytidectomy. Clin Plast Surg 1978;5(1):109–19.
5. Muenker R. Problems and variation in cervicofacial rhytidectomy. Facial Plast Surg 1992;8(1):33–51.
6. Adamson P, Moran ML. Complications of cervicofacial rhytidectomy. Facial Plast Surg Clin North Am 1993;112:257–70.
7. McKinney P, Katrana DJ. Prevention of injury to the great auricular nerve during rhytidectomy. Plast Reconstr Surg 1977;59:525–9.
8. Liebman EP, Webster RC, Gaul JR, et al. The marginal mandibular nerve in rhytidectomy and liposuction surgery. Arch Otolaryngol Head Neck Surg 1988;114:179–81.
9. Bitner JB, Friedman O, Farrior RT, et al. Direct submentoplasty for neck rejuvenation. Arch Facial Plast Surg 2007;9(3):194–200.
10. Maliniak JW. Is the surgical restoration of the aged face justified? Indications, method of repair, end result. Med J Rec 1932;135:321–4.
11. Johnson JB. The problem of the aging face. Plast Reconstr Surg 1955;15:117–21.
12. Adamson JE, Horton CE, Crawford HH. The surgical correction of the "turkey gobbler" deformity. Plast Reconstr Surg 1964;34:598–605.
13. Henderson J, O'Niell T, Logan A. Direct anterior neck skin excision for cervicomental laxity. Aesthetic Plast Surg 2010;34:299–305.
14. Cronin TD, Biggs TM. The T-Z-plasty for the male "turkey gobbler" neck. Plast Reconstr Surg 1971; 47:534–8.
15. Biggs TM. The T-Z-plasty for the male "turkey gobbler" neck. Plast Reconstr Surg 1980;65(2):238.
16. Ehlert TK, Thomas JR, Becker FF Jr. Submental W-plasty for correction of "turkey gobbler" deformity. Arch Otolaryngol Head Neck Surg 1990; 116:714–7.
17. Farrior RT, Jarchow RC, Farrior EH. Surgical principles in face-lift: instructional courses, vol. 3. St Louis (MO): Mosby-Year Book; 1990. p. 215–26.

The Extended SMAS Approach to Neck Rejuvenation

Stephen W. Perkins, MD[a,b,*], Heather H. Waters, MD[b]

KEYWORDS

- Facelift • Facial rejuventation • Neck contour • Neck lift • Neck rejuvenation • Platysmaplasty

KEY POINTS

- The key to substantial, long-lasting improvement in rhytidectomy is to manage the neck adequately.
- The Kelly clamp platysmal imbrication is the foundation for an improved cervicomental angle.
- Skeletal augmentation and adjunctive procedures can further enhance the overall outcome.
- Poor incision planning with obvious scars and an altered hairline are not easily camouflaged, and are a telltale sign of rhytidectomy.
- Overly aggressive liposuction can lead to dermal banding and visible submandibular glands.

 Videos of submental skin elevation, Perkins platysmaplasty technique, and SMAS elevation and suspension accompany this article at http://www.facialplastic.theclinics.com/

INTRODUCTION

Determining the patient's aesthetic concerns is the foundation of a thoughtful discussion on rejuvenation procedures. Patients requesting a facelift may specifically request correction of facial skin laxity/ptosis and jowl formation, whereas others may primarily desire neck improvement with reduction of submental lipoptosis, relaxation of platysmal bands, and sharpening of an oblique cervicomental angle. This latter group may also appropriately ask for a facelift with different goals, or request only a necklift. They may even say, "I don't want a facelift, all I want is a necklift." In reality, rejuvenation of the neck and lower face are accomplished together.

The fundamental concept of rhytidectomy is based on certain anatomic relationships of the tissues. The elasticity and condition of the overlying skin, including its degree of photodamage and rhytid formation, is important. The relationship with the underlying subcutaneous tissue, including the vector of descent as a result of gravity, true ptosis, or abnormal accumulation and distribution of fat must be noted.

Facial musculature is enveloped by continuous fascia that extends to the preparotid region. This fascia, which is contiguous with the platysma muscle of the neck, is the superficial muscular aponeurotic system (SMAS) (Fig. 1). In the neck anteriorly, the platysma muscle may or may not be interdigitated to form a connected sling depending on age. Often, there is a laxity and dehiscence of the anterior borders of the platysma muscle, creating banding in the neck. It is the very nature and the existence of this SMAS layer that allows for a deeper plane of facelifting surgery than was performed in the original rhytidectomy procedures of the past. It is easily demonstrable that lifting and pulling the SMAS layer with its integral attachment to the platysma muscle and

Nothing to Disclose.

[a] Department of Otolaryngology – Head and Neck Surgery, Indiana University School of Medicine, 702 Riley Hospital Drive, Indianapolis, IN 46202, USA; [b] Meridian Plastic Surgery Center, 170 West 106th Street, Indianapolis, IN 46290–0970, USA

* Corresponding author. Meridian Plastic Surgery Center, 170 West 106th Street, Indianapolis, IN 46290–0970.
E-mail address: sperkski@gmail.com

Facial Plast Surg Clin N Am 22 (2014) 253–268
http://dx.doi.org/10.1016/j.fsc.2014.01.010
1064-7406/14/$ – see front matter © 2014 Elsevier Inc. All rights reserved.

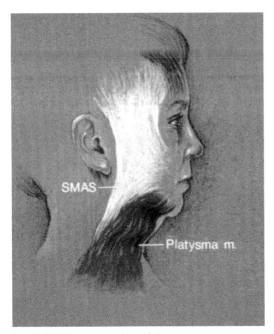

Fig. 1. SMAS connected to platysma.

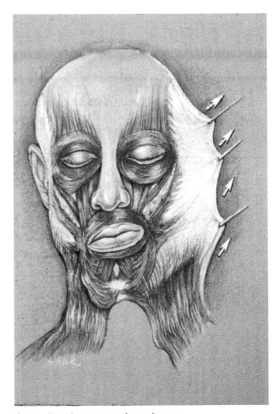

Fig. 2. SMAS connected to platysma.

midfacial muscles lifts and repositions the skin in the same fashion without undue tension on the skin edges. A superior and posterior vector of pull of this fascia repositions the facial and neck tissues in a more youthful position (**Fig. 2**). The visible effect of gravity on these anatomic tissues is directly countered and improved by the facelifting procedures. It is the senior author's practice to perform a standard platysmaplasty on all patients, in addition to the extended SMAS rhytidectomy to achieve a "sling" in the cervicomental area, which can then be used for posterior tightening of the skin–SMAS–platysma.

TREATMENT GOALS AND PLANNED OUTCOMES

The examination begins with a general assessment of the patient's overall health, facial features, and symmetry. Critical in analyzing patients presenting for rhytidectomy includes those items listed in **Box 1**. Although all factors are important, those directly related to the neck are most critical and ultimately lead to the success of the extended SMAS rhytidectomy. Together, these factors are used to grade the patient preoperatively into one of three categories per the senior author's classification system. A type I rhytidectomy patient demonstrates good skin elasticity, minimal jowling, minimal to no lipoptosis, early cheek and neck skin laxity, and minor platysmal laxity or banding (**Fig. 3**). Most common is the type II rhytidectomy

patient who presents with moderate facial and neck skin ptosis, clear jowling, moderate lipoptosis, and heavier platysmal banding with an obtuse cervicomental angle (**Fig. 4**). The type III rhytidectomy patient, including most men, has heavy cheeks, prominent jowling with frequent prejowl grooves, loss of mandibular definition, significant platysmal bands with large amounts of lipoptosis, and absent cervicomental angle or convexity of the neck (**Figs. 5** and **6**). This grading system is directly related to the expected amount of surgical work and intervention to create a long-lasting and pleasing neck contour. Additionally, the underlying skeletal structure should be noted, because a low hyoid position portends difficulty creating a sharp cervicomental angle (**Fig. 7**). Moreover, a chin or

---

Box 1
Examination criteria

Submental and submandibular skin redundancy

Lipoptosis

Platysmal banding

Midface ptosis and hollowing

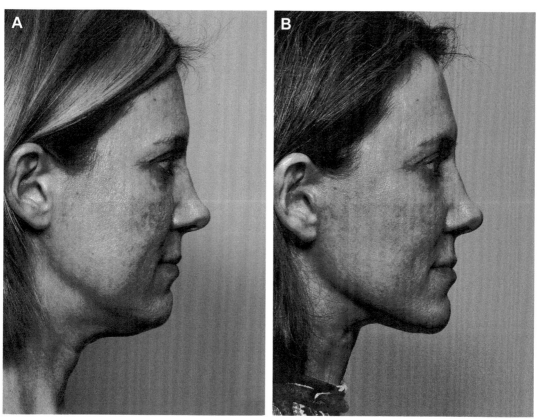

Fig. 3. (*A*) Type I rhytidectomy patient, preoperatively. (*B*) Type I rhytidectomy patient, postoperatively.

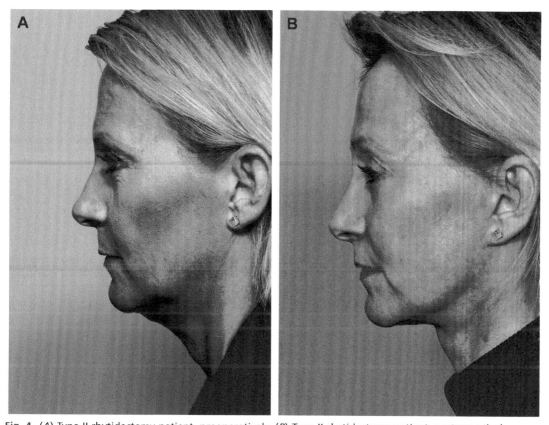

Fig. 4. (*A*) Type II rhytidectomy patient, preoperatively. (*B*) Type II rhytidectomy patient, postoperatively.

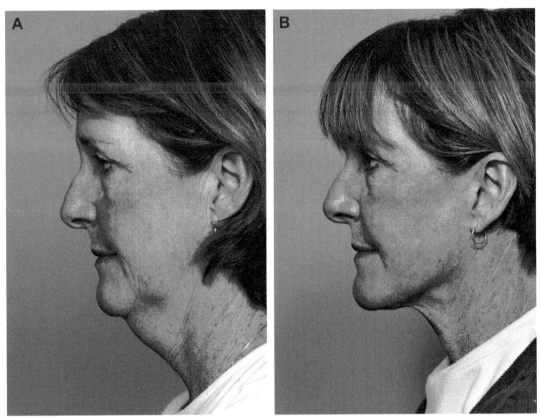

Fig. 5. (*A*) Type III rhytidectomy patient, preoperatively. (*B*) Type III rhytidectomy patient, postoperatively.

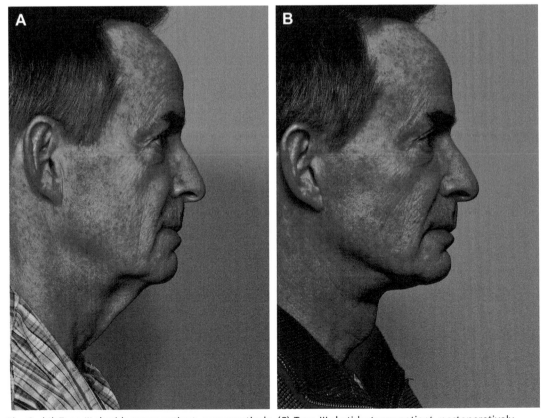

Fig. 6. (*A*) Type III rhytidectomy patient, preoperatively. (*B*) Type III rhytidectomy patient, postoperatively.

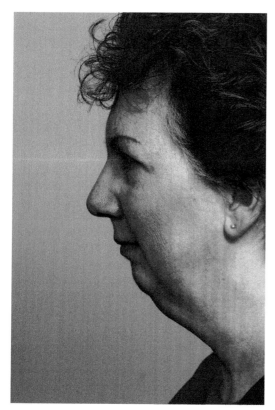

Fig. 7. Weak chin, low hyoid in poor facelift candidate.

prejowl implant can improve the structure and overall result in select cases. Lastly, the periorbital, perioral, brow, and midface should be evaluated for adjuvant procedures during rhytidectomy.

For motivated patients with realistic expectations, the extended SMAS rhytidectomy in concert with a submentoplasty is warranted. Age-related ptotic facial and neck skin, rhytids, jowl formation, platysmal banding, and lipoptosis are all indications for this surgical intervention.

Most absolute contraindications for rhytidectomy are factors that compromise wound healing of the large facial skin flap (**Box 2**). Relative contraindications include characteristics that can lead to a less than satisfied patient. In particular, a low hyoid position limits the ability recreate an acute neckline because of the underlying suprahyoid strap muscles obstructing the placement of a high, tight platysmaplasty. A weak mandible makes enhancing the transition between the face and neck a challenge even with liposuction and tightening of the heavy overlying skin. Similarly, ptotic submandibular glands can be misinterpreted as persistent lipoptosis in the neck, and detract from a smooth lateral neck contour. If present, each of these findings should be communicated to the patient so that expectations can be

managed appropriately. Some surgeons advocate partial or total excision of the submandibular glands for maximum cosmetic benefit. The senior author does not perform this procedure or believe it is an appropriate "cosmetic" indication. Lastly, a patient currently experiencing a period of high stress or a major life-changing event may be prompted to surgical intervention for the wrong reasons. This may lead to an unhappy patient when facial rejuvenation does not fulfill their goals.

PREOPERATIVE PLANNING AND PREPARATION

With the patient's desires known and the examination complete, final planning begins for the extended SMAS rhytidectomy with submentoplasty. Adjuvant procedures including neurotoxins, facial fillers, skeletal augmentation, skin resurfacing, and management of the forehead, midface, and eyes are also discussed at this time. Next, digital photographs are captured to document the patient's preoperative condition and are used as a medium for digital imaging. Standard preoperative photographic views for facelift surgery include the full-face frontal view, and full-face left and right oblique views, and left and right lateral views. One may choose a close-up perioral photograph, and a close-up showing more detail of the submental neck tissues. A close-up view of each auricle, with hair pulled behind the ears, earrings removed, and all photographs taken in a Frankfort horizontal line, is imperative. This is routinely used as a tool to further communicate a realistic representation of the expected result. Often, this is a powerful tool to demonstrate to the patient the dramatic improvement that can be expected in the neckline and jowl/jawline. A patient rarely realizes and appreciates the degree of aging changes visible from their profile. This greatly helps the patient visualize and prepare for the postoperative change. If the patient is satisfied, a date is scheduled, routine laboratory work is ordered, and the appropriate cardiac examinations and imaging are obtained. Routinely, prescriptions are given for antibiotics, analgesics, antiemetics, anxiolytics, and sleep aids at this time. Any herbals or pharmaceuticals that increase the patient's risk of hemorrhage are discontinued in a timely manner before surgery. Finally, verbal and written instructions for the perioperative period are given to the patient.

PATIENT POSITIONING

In the preoperative holding area, the markings are made with a surgical pen for the rhytidectomy and for additional procedures (**Fig. 8**). The preauricular marking is carefully planned so as not to distort the temporal hair tuft, because it routinely stops at the inferior extent of the tuft or no higher than the upper anterior helical insertion. It incorporates a posttragal course as it is continued inferiorly in all women, and in some men. One variation in the male facelift patient with preauricular hair-bearing skin is an incision that is gently curved in the preauricular area in what is often a preexisting preauricular crease. This incision should not be entirely straight; rather, it should be a distance away from the incisura and in front of the tragus. One must leave a non–hair-bearing portion of skin when moving the bearded skin or hair-bearing skin posteriorly and superiorly (**Fig. 9**). However, for many aging men the preauricular region bears thin or sparse hair follicles and a posttragal incision may be used. The marking then continues around the ear lobule and is placed above the postauricular sulcus on the posterior surface of the concha. As the marking reaches the level of the helical

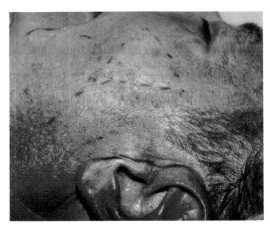
Fig. 9. Typical incision for a man with a beard, preserving non–hair-bearing preauricular skin.

insertion, it is directed posteriorly with a gentle curve along and into the hairline. Lastly, a 3-cm marking for the submentoplasty is made in the submental crease, and the hair is twirled and taped to remove it from the operative field.

After an appropriate level of anesthesia is achieved, the patient is appropriately positioned in the supine position and the incision sites of the face and neck are infiltrated with 1% lidocaine with 1:50,000 epinephrine. The areas of undermining are also infiltrated with a combination of 1% lidocaine with 1:100,000 epinephrine, and 0.5% lidocaine with 1:100,000 epinephrine. If neurotoxin or filler is to be injected, it is done at this time. The patient is then prepared and draped in the usual sterile manner while vasoconstriction and analgesia from the anesthetic take effect.

PROCEDURAL APPROACH

Initial treatment of the neck involves correction of the jowl, submandibular, and submental lipoptosis. The submentoplasty is initiated by making the submental skin incision with a #15 Bard Parker blade. A short flap is then elevated with Metzenbaum scissors just beneath the skin in the middle of the fat layer or subcutaneous tissues, and hemostasis is obtained with bipolar cautery. Through this incision, either a chin or prejowl implant can be placed without difficulty at this time. Otherwise, a circular 3-mm liposuction cannula with three openings on one side is used to make radial tunnels throughout the anterior neck within the subcutaneous plane (**Fig. 10**). No suction is applied initially, creating the tunnels from the submental area across the mandibular margin into the jowl region, down to the anterior border of the sternocleidomastoid muscle (SCM) and across the cervical mental angle to the area of the thyroid

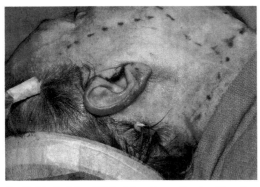
Fig. 8. Typical facelift incision for patient with a low sideburn tuft of hair.

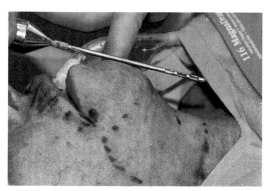

Fig. 10. A 3-mm three-opening liposuction cannula.

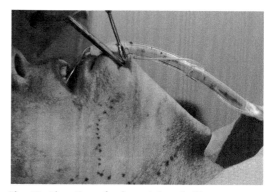

Fig. 11. Elevation of submental neck skin.

cartilage. This is done in a fanlike fashion from one jowl across the neck to the opposite jowl. After the initial tunnels are created, 1 atm of suction is applied to the same cannula and it is used to remove the excess fat. The nondominant hand lifts and guides the cannula with the opening always directed away from the overlying dermis. Particular attention is given to avoid overzealous liposuctioning and subsequent dimpling in the jowl regions. Depending on the amount of liposuction required in the submental and submandibular neck, a larger liposuction cannula may be required. A 4- or 6-mm flat cannula with one opening on the inferior surface of the cannula is then required to obtain adequate removal and contouring. Bimanual palpation is required to determine the symmetry and equality of the removal of the fat. Leaving a thin layer of subcutaneous fat is required to give supple skin contour. Caution should be exercised in terms of not being overly aggressive in performing liposuction across the cervical mental angle, because this has the potential for creating dermal injury and subdermal scarring, with late development of banding. Aggressive liposuction in the submental area also may contribute to a cobra deformity.

Direct subcutaneous elevation is then performed to elevate the skin from the platysma muscle. This is performed in a wide fashion, usually extending to the anterior border of the sternocleidomastoid and past the cervical mental angle with Metzenbaum scissors (Fig. 11). Meticulous hemostasis is then achieved with a protected bayonet-style bipolar cautery. This allows the surgeon to directly view the remaining lipoptosis beneath the platysma muscle and observe the redundancy and laxity of the anterior platysma bands. Their dehiscence is readily visible.

Next, using a curved Kelly clamp, the excess loose fat and platysma that is easily grasped in the midline down to the level of the hyoid bone, is clamped (Fig. 12). This may include some superficial fat, some loose anterior platysma, and some subplatysmal fat. Once clamped, the redundancy is cauterized, cut, and sutured with a 3-0 Vicryl (Ethicon, Somerville, NJ) suture in a sequential manner until the entire clamped portion of tissue has been removed, leaving a tightly imbricated platysma corset to support the submental area (Fig. 13). In most men, and in women with heavier necks, 3.0 Tevdek permanent sutures (Teleflex Medical, Research Triangle Park, NC, USA) are added. After a firm muscular corset is created, a small wedge of platysma muscle is excised for a sharper cervicomental angle (Fig. 14). The remainder of the facelift skin undermining is accomplished from the posterior position. Redundancy of skin in the submental area is determined at the end of the operation after tightening of the bilateral preauricular and postauricular skin in a superior posterior direction.

Rhytidectomy is initiated by incising the postauricular markings with a #15 Bard Parker blade from the lobule into the scalp. In the scalp, the incision is beveled to avoid injury to adjacent hair follicles, and subsequent flap elevation remains deep to the follicles to avoid postoperative alopecia in the hair-bearing region. The flap elevation is

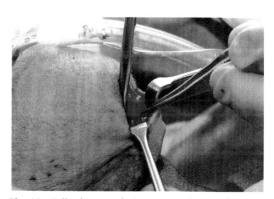

Fig. 12. Kelly clamp technique: grasp loose submental soft tissues with anterior platysmal borders.

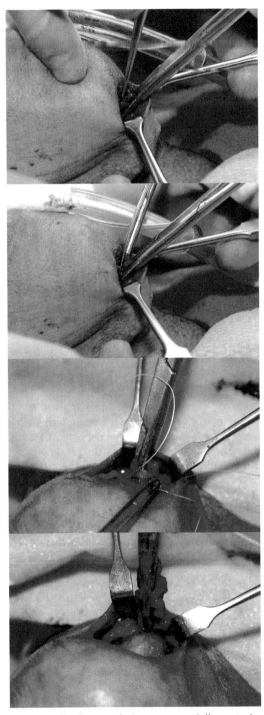

Fig. 13. Kelly clamp technique: sequentially cauterize and cut the clamped soft tissue and platysma, followed by suture imbrication of the anterior platysmal borders in midline and excision of the clamped soft tissues.

aided by the use of nonpenetrating towel clamps for traction and performed with a scalpel dissecting just on top of the SCM fascia. Once this short segment is elevated, complete hemostasis is again obtained with bipolar cautery. The anterior incision is then made, as marked previously, and beveled appropriately while adjacent to the temporal hair tuft. Again, nonpenetrating towel clamps are placed on the temporal portion of the flap for traction and a small area is elevated in the preauricular area with the scalpel. This is followed by meticulous hemostasis with bipolar cautery.

Using the Kahn facelift dissecting scissors, the remaining posterior skin flap is elevated, first with countertraction provided by the nondominant hand grasping the towel clamps, and countertraction is maintained on the cheek of the neck with the taut fingers of the assistant. Further traction on the distal flap is provided by an assistant, which greatly improves exposure during elevation. The scissors, which are slightly blunted and have an outward bevel, are used in an advancing, spreading motion to achieve flap elevation (Fig. 15). Thin, intervening bridges of fat and dermal connective tissue are then sharply released with the partially opened scissors. Once completely elevated posteriorly and in continuity with the previously undermined neck flap, retractors are placed and hemostasis is obtained with bipolar cautery.

The anterior skin flap is then elevated in a similar manner using Kahn facelift scissors in the subcutaneous plane. After elevation, the anterior, posterior, and neck flaps are in continuity allowing for complete visualization of the SMAS-platysma sling (Fig. 16). The anterior extent of this dissection is dictated by the patient's anatomy, but it does not extend medial to the nasolabial fold. Meticulous hemostasis is again obtained before performing the extended SMAS flap.

Using the zygomatic arch as a landmark, the SMAS is incised with a #15 Bard Parker blade in a semilunar fashion from the arch to anterior border of the SCM (Fig. 17). The flap is then elevated medially with a combination of sharp and blunt dissection anterior to the parotid (Fig. 18). As the dissection continues, the masseter muscle, zygomatic major muscle, and the distal facial nerve branches are visualized. Complete hemostasis is required for safe dissection, and care must be taken to avoid injury to the facial nerve. The extent of the sub-SMAS elevation is adequate when firm traction on the SMAS flap gives the desired amount of correction (Fig. 19). There is no absolute distance, because this varies depending on each patient's tissues and SMAS stability. Once obtained, the SMAS is then secured to maintain this result (Fig. 20).

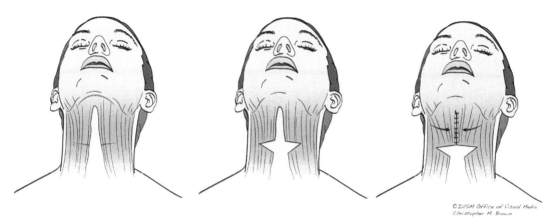

Fig. 14. Wedge excision of platysma at cervicomental angle after plastysmaplasty. © 2013 IUSM Office of Visual Media, C. M. Brown.

SMAS imbrication begins with preauricular suspension along a posterior-superior vector (**Fig. 21**). This is then secured near the zygomatic root with a buried 0 Vicryl suture. Once placed, the SMAS is partially divided for a secondary vector of suspension. The inferior portion is then anchored posteriorly with another 0 Vicryl to the mastoid periosteum just behind the ear lobule (**Fig. 22**). The SMAS is not excised, but advanced over the superior and posterior fascial tissues and is used as a "sling" suspension. The only SMAS that is excised is a small portion in the immediate preauricular region. Additional, 3-0 Monocryl (Ethicon) sutures are used to further support the SMAS flap and smooth its edges. Occasionally, 3-0 Tevdek (Teleflex Medical, Research Triangle Park, NC, USA) sutures are necessary to suspend heavier flaps. Once the SMAS is secure in its new location, all the tension of the closure rests on this deeper tissue and allows the skin to be closed without strain on the wound edges. This avoids widening of the scar and suture tract formation that would otherwise occur.

Next, to reposition the preauricular skin flap, it is first advanced posteriorly and slightly superiorly. First, the posterior flap is elevated posteriorly, then rotated superiorly, and suspension staples are placed with particular attention to align the posterior hairline properly (**Fig. 23**). It is then further secured in the preauricular area with suspension staples placed in key positions. Following this, the posterior flap redundancy is removed and the scalp is closed immediately with surgical staples. The skin flap is then tailored to cradle the ear lobule in a tension-free manner. This is a critical step to avoid a postoperative pixie or satyr ear deformity. The anterior skin flap edge is then trimmed to mirror both the anterior lobule and helical insertion. Before closure, a 7-mm closed suction drain is placed in a dependent position and brought out through a separate stab incision posteriorly (**Fig. 24**).

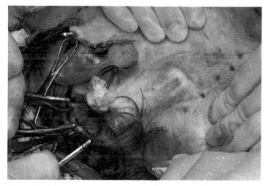

Fig. 15. Undermining postauricular neck skin with beveled facelift scissors with advance-and-spread technique.

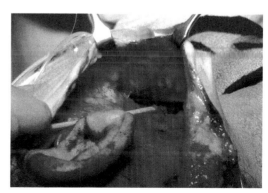

Fig. 16. Postauricular flap elevation within subcutaneous fat.

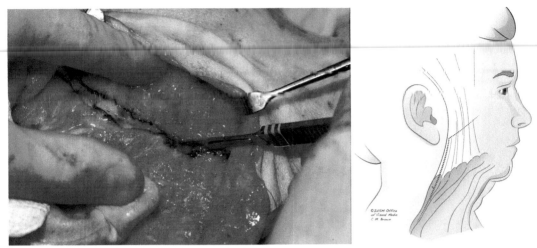

Fig. 17. Incising the SMAS.   © 2013 IUSM Office of Visual Media, C. M. Brown.

After obtaining hemostasis, several 5-0 Monocryl sutures are used to reapproximate the contoured flap, and two 6-0 Ethilon (Ethicon) sutures placed in the lobule to maintain the tucked position. Next, the distal portion of the tragal flap is thinned of the subcutaneous tissue and left slightly redundant to help avoid blunting or anterior displacement of the underlying cartilage. The closure is then completed with removal of the suspension staples and placement of a 5-0 Plain Gut suture in a running, locking fashion.

The procedure is then performed on the contralateral side in an identical manner. After both sides have been completed and closed, the submental incision is trimmed of redundant skin and similarly closed with 5-0 Plain Gut sutures in a running, locking fashion. Once completed, resurfacing procedures, if indicated, are performed. Although a resurfacing procedure is never performed directly over the undermined portion of the preauricular or neck skin because of the possibility of vascular

compromise, the perioral area and deeper lip rhytids are frequently treated. Lastly, the drains are attached to closed bulb suction. An antibiotic ointment is applied to a nonadherent dressing that is placed in the preauricular and postauricular regions. Four-by-four sterile gauzes are placed over the undermined areas and under the chin. This is followed by a loose circumferential dressing including ABD pads and held in place with a minimally constrictive wrap of Kerlix (Covidien, Mansfield, MA, USA) (**Fig. 25**). Care is taken not to apply excess pressure to the undermined skin flaps (Videos 1–3).

POTENTIAL COMPLICATIONS AND MANAGEMENT

An expanding postsurgical hematoma is a surgical emergency and requires early recognition and return to the operating room under anesthesia for evacuation and hemostasis. Luckily, these rarely

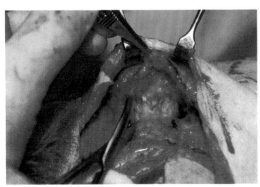

Fig. 18. Elevation of the preauricular SMAS with Metzenbaum scissors.

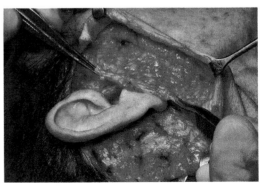

Fig. 19. Advancement of the undermined SMAS before suspension and imbrication.

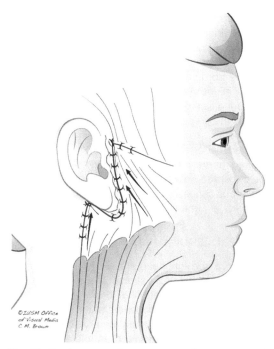

Fig. 20. Dual vector advancement and suspension of the extended SMAS flap. © 2013 IUSM Office of Visual Media, C. M. Brown.

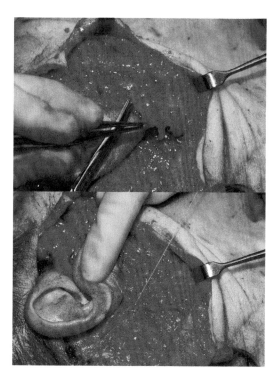

Fig. 22. Splitting the SMAS/platysma at the lobule with suspension of posterior slip of platysma-SMAS to the mastoid periosteum.

occur, and if treated appropriately, do not lead to adverse outcomes. More frequently, small, nonexpanding hematomas and seromas can be easily treated with needle aspiration, continued antibiotic coverage, a firm dressing, and close observation. Rarely, a small opening and insertion of a Penrose drain is required for large persistent seromas. Infections are unlikely unless flap perfusion is compromised or a fluid collection is present. Supportive care with treatment of the underlying cause and aggressive antibiotic management are required. Wound opening with evacuation is rarely required.

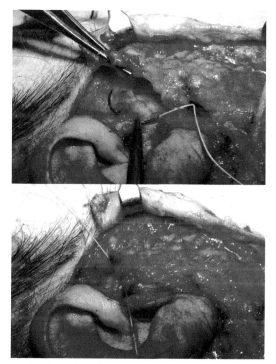

Fig. 21. Superior advancement and suspension of SMAS to the posterior zygomatic periosteum.

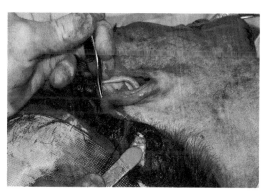

Fig. 23. Posterior draping of the skin flap requires alignment of the occipital hairline.

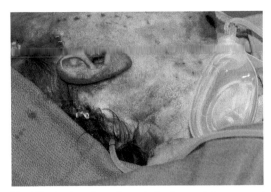

Fig. 24. A closed suction drain is used to prevent serohematomas.

Skin loss from any of these conditions, or other patient factors, such as continued smoking, can be problematic. Poor early postoperative perfusion may be improved with warm compresses, massage, and/or nitroglycerin ointment, in addition to treatment of the underlying cause, if possible. Ultimately, mild epidermolysis usually heals quickly, whereas full-thickness loss may remain unsightly for many months and lead to scarring of varying significance. This almost exclusively occurs in patients who smoke in the immediate postoperative period, or those who did not quit, as instructed. In full-thickness skin defects, the eschar should be allowed to slough spontaneously during wound contraction, and attempts at removal should be avoided.

Persistent edema and mild irregularities are relatively common and can be managed well with local triamcinolone injections as needed. Occasionally, mild hypervascularity is seen after rhytidectomy or after steroids injections but, given adequate time, usually resolve spontaneously. Alternatively, asymmetries or inadequately treated areas may require a touch-up procedure if a period of watchful waiting does not resolve the problem.

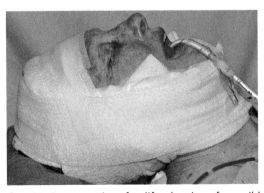

Fig. 25. Postoperative facelift dressing for mild compression.

Temporary sensory loss is expected, and each patient is instructed on this normal postoperative sequela. In nearly every case, complete return of sensation occurs, but may take a variable length of time from several weeks to 1 year. Permanent nerve injuries are also possible, and should be managed as any other neural injury. This usually involves the greater auricular nerve. In each of these conditions, reassurance is required but, with proper management and reapproximation of the injured nerve, complete return of sensation can be expected. Injury to the facial nerve is reported in various series, but has not occurred in the senior author's experience.

POSTPROCEDURAL CARE

Overnight, the light head dressing and closed suction drains remain. Elevation of the head of the bed and frequent application of cool compresses is recommended. The patient should rest the first night and begin ambulation the next day. The patient's diet can be advanced as tolerated. Antibiotics, analgesics, anxiolytics, antiemetics, and sleep aids are taken as instructed to maintain comfort and minimize risk of infection. On postoperative day 1, the patient is re-evaluated and the dressing and drains are removed. Wound care is performed and demonstrated until the patient has a full understanding of the postoperative instructions. A lighter, mildly constrictive wrap is applied to the neck for the next 24 hours. The second postoperative day, the patient no longer needs the dressing, and begins washing their hair daily. Light activity, continued head elevation, and frequent cool compresses are recommended. On postoperative day 7, the patient returns for removal of all but the lobule sutures and re-evaluation of the results. On postoperative day 10, lobule sutures are removed, and a make-up and skincare session is performed by our medical estheticians. The patient is instructed regarding appropriate makeup coverage for any residual ecchymosis and is given a full skincare lesson. The makeup artist introduces appropriate moisturizers, cosmetics, and sunscreens, and informs the patient about future appropriate skincare practices to maintain the facelift results.

REHABILITATION AND RECOVERY

At 3 weeks, normal activity can be resumed. The patient returns for follow-up appointments at 1 week, 3 months, 6 months, and 1 year, or longer, to assess the results and confirm patient satisfaction (**Figs. 26–29**). In the second to fourth week, the patient often requires emotional support,

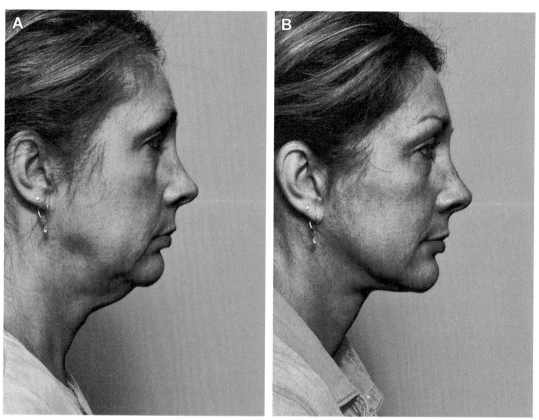

Fig. 26. (A) Preoperative, lateral view. (B) Five months postoperative, lateral view.

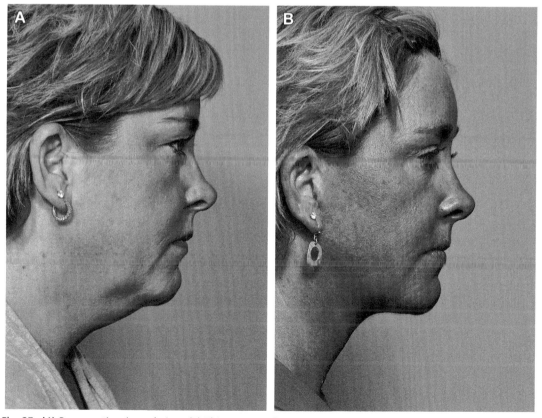

Fig. 27. (A) Preoperative, lateral view. (B) Thirteen months postoperative, lateral view.

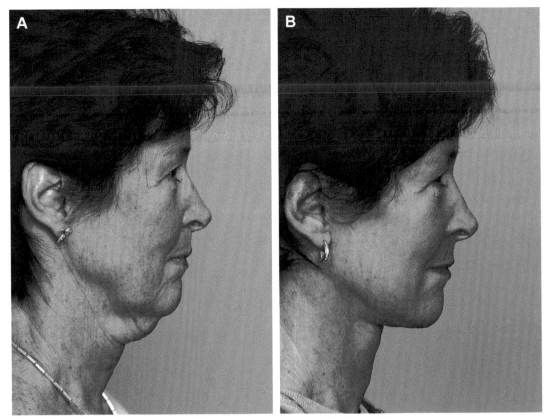

Fig. 28. (*A*) Preoperative, lateral view. (*B*) Four months postoperative, lateral view.

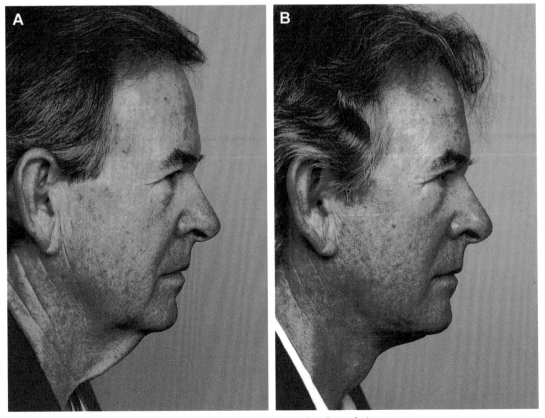

Fig. 29. (*A*) Preoperative, lateral view. (*B*) One year postoperative, lateral view.

Table 1
Change in mentocervical angle

	Preoperatively	6 mo	1 y	5 y
Mentocervical angle	113.65	94.17	96.42	94.67
Change in angle		19.98[a]	19.97[a]	20.04[a]

[a] *P*<.001.

Data from Brobst R, Sufyan A, Perkins SW. Kelly clamp technique for submental plastysmaplasty: evaluation of long-term outcomes. In press.

because adjustment is still being made to the new appearance, and reassimilating to work or social activities. Many of the postoperative sensations being experienced, and minor healing variabilities that the patient was informed would occur, have been forgotten and reassurance is needed that everything is progressing as expected. Continuous reaffirmation of postoperative instructions and expectations is critical to the happiness of these elective cosmetic surgical patients. Your office should be a place they feel comfortable calling, and returning to, in this immediate postoperative time. Patients must feel that you are there for them, to answer questions and reassure them. This is critical to their long-term satisfaction. For long-term follow-up, it is important that you intervene if there is any tendency toward hypertrophic healing in the postauricular areas. Intralesional steroids may occasionally be required to settle down a slightly thickened postauricular scar. In addition, at the 4- to 6-week postoperative period, if the patient is going to experience some temporary surgical alopecia in the hair-bearing areas,

he or she needs complete reassurance that these hair follicles will regenerate hair shafts and that within 4 to 6 months all of the hair will grow back. The patient further needs reassurance throughout the first 3 to 6 months that hypersensitivities and neuresthesias are completely normal and part of the healing process.

OUTCOMES

As patients are followed throughout the first year postoperatively, it is inevitable that they will experience a certain degree of rebound relaxation in the superficial tissues of the face and neck. This is despite excellent efforts on the part of the surgeon to give them a long-term tightened jaw and neckline. This is very much a function of their inherent hereditary loss of elasticity, which occasionally requires a small procedure to improve the overall results. Submental tuck-up procedures to correct small residual submental bands or fullness may be required in up to 5% of patients, depending on their preoperative condition and skin elasticity.

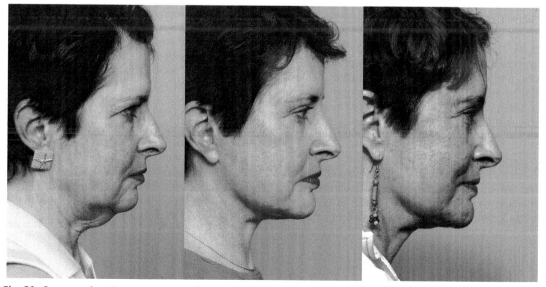

Fig. 30. Preoperative, 1 year postoperative, 6 years postoperative, lateral view.

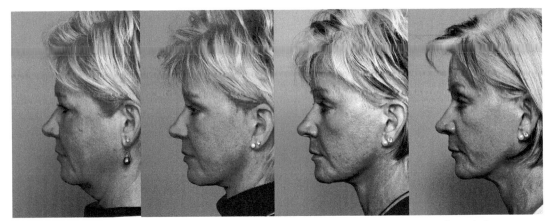

Fig. 31. Preoperative, 1 year postoperative, 5 years postoperative, 11 years postoperative, lateral view.

This should be offered to them as part of the overall facelift experience and may be necessary despite excellent technique. More rarely, the jowl, because of its fullness and presurgical condition, reverts enough to require a cheek tuck-up. This is the area most likely to disappoint patients in terms of overall results. Whatever area needs to be addressed, must be to achieve the long-term results and satisfaction they had expected.

The senior author has recently reviewed his efficacy in the management of the aging neck in patients undergoing standard platysmaplasty with extended SMAS rhytidectomy. Mentocervical angle measurements were obtained from preoperative and postoperative photographs in a retrospective review of 840 patients. A two-tailed paired t-test revealed that the postoperative angles at 6 months, 1 year, and 5 years continued to demonstrate significant improvement compared with the preoperative angles t (34) = 12.085 ($P<.001$) (**Table 1**). These improvements were seen for all groups, including facelift types I to III and those classified as having a hypoplastic mentum or low hyoid position. The long-term experience of the senior author demonstrates that the use of the Kelly clamp technique in platysmaplasty results in an effective and reliable method of managing the aging neck.

SUMMARY

The senior author's fundamental technique has changed very little over the past 15 to 20 years. It has provided patients with excellent, natural,

lasting results, and overall satisfaction (**Figs. 30** and **31**).

SUPPLEMENTARY DATA

Supplementary data related to this article can be found online at http://dx.doi.org/10.1016/j.fsc.2014.01.010.

FURTHER READINGS

Baker SR. Tri-plane rhytidectomy. Arch Otolaryngol Head Neck Surg 1997;123:1167–72.

Hamra ST. The deep plane rhytidectomy. Plast Reconstr Surg 1990;86:53–61.

Kamer FM. One hundred consecutive deep plane face lifts. Arch Otolaryngol Head Neck Surg 1996;122:17–22.

Koch BB, Perkins SW. Simultaneous rhytidectomy and full-face carbon dioxide laser resurfacing: a case series and meta-analysis. Arch Facial Plast Surg 2002;4:227–33.

McCollough EG, Perkins SW, Langsdon PR. SMAS suspension rhytidectomy, rationale and long term experience. Arch Otolaryngol Head Neck Surg 1989;115:228–34.

Mitz V, Peyronie M. The superficial musculo-aponeurotic system (SMAS) in the parotid and cheek area. Plast Reconstr Surg 1976;58:80–8.

Perkins SW, Williams JD, MacDonald K, et al. Prevention of seromas and hematomas following facelift surgery with the use of postoperative vacuum drains. Arch Otolaryngol Head Neck Surg 1997;123:743–5.

Skoog T. Plastic surgery: new methods and refinements. Philadelphia: W.B. Saunders; 1974.

The Deep-Plane Approach to Neck Rejuvenation

Neil A. Gordon, MD[a,b], Stewart I. Adam, MD[a],*

KEYWORDS

- Neck rejuvenation • Deep plane • Facelift • Rhytidectomy • Neck lift • Aging face
- Platysma muscle

KEY POINTS

- Neck changes are often the motivator for seeking treatment of the aging face.
- The platysma muscle/superficial muscular aponeurotic system/galea are the continuous superficial cervical fascia, encompassing most of the facial and neck fat. This superficial soft-tissue envelope is poorly anchored to the face and neck.
- Facial aging is mainly due to gravity's long-term effects on the superficial soft-tissue envelope, with more subtle effects on the deeper structural compartments, manifesting in soft-tissue redundancy throughout the face and neck.
- The deep cervical fascia binds the structural aspects of the face and neck, and covers the facial nerve and buccal fat pad.
- The deep plane is the embryologic cleavage plane between these fascial layers and is the logical place for midfacial dissection, which allows access to the buccal fat pad for treatment of jowling.
- Soft-tissue mobilization is maximized in deep-plane midface dissections. Because the superficial soft-tissue envelope is continuous from the midface to the neck, this technique creates the best opportunity for reestablishing proper neck contour.
- Flap advancement creates tension only at the fascia level and is the optimal technique for revision rhytidectomy.
- The lack of skin tension in the deep-plane advancement flap allows natural, long-lasting outcomes, and is resistant to complications.

 A video of a complete extended deep-plane midface lift with platysma tightening accompanies the article.

INTRODUCTION

Change in neck contour is the most common complaint that motivates a potential patient to consider a rhytidectomy. Patients desire a youthful appearance, bolstered by a well-defined neck and clear jawline. Of all facial changes associated with aging, loss of neck contour and jawline are most often associated with advanced aging.

The principal goals in neck rejuvenation, which were defined by Ellenbogen and Karlin[1] in 1980, include creating a distinct mandibular border, subhyoid depression, thyroid bulge, a distinct border to the sternocleidomastoid muscle, and a cervicomental angle of 105° to 120°. Whereas the primary and often sole cause of blunted neck contour in younger patients is excess fat deposition, this

Funding Sources: None.

Conflict of Interest: None.

[a] Section of Otolaryngology, Head and Neck Surgery, Department of Surgery, Yale University School of Medicine, New Haven, CT 06510, USA; [b] New England Surgical Center, The Retreat at Split Rock, 539 Danbury Road, Wilton, CT 06897, USA

* Corresponding author. Yale Physicians Building, 4th Floor, 800 Howard Avenue, New Haven, CT 06510.

E-mail address: stewart.adam@yale.edu

Facial Plast Surg Clin N Am 22 (2014) 269–284

http://dx.doi.org/10.1016/j.fsc.2014.01.003

process is not the main factor in the aging neck. Gravity's lifetime effects on facial soft tissue, combined with facial skeletal changes and fat deposition, are the key factors that dictate neck aging. The proportions each factor contributes are based on case-specific age and anatomy.

In general, gravity's long-term downward pull on the poorly anchored facial superficial soft-tissue envelope is the central component in facial/neck aging. This process is confirmed by both facial palpation and intraoperative rhytidectomy views of the excessive, redundant facial soft tissue following sub–superficial muscular aponeurotic system (SMAS) facial dissection and flap mobilization (**Fig. 1**). Moreover, facial skeletal remodeling causes certain aging changes, specifically around the periorbital, pyriform, and mandible regions.[2] This process provides an explanation for the loosening of both fascial and muscular attachments, leading to pseudoherniation of fat pads and ptosis of these muscular structures. In addition, loss of mandibular height is responsible for the abrupt change in jawline and neck contour with advanced age.[2] Fat deposition can be a contributing factor to a suboptimal neck contour at any age.

Viewing the neck in layers, most of the changes resulting from skin, fat, and muscular aging are confined to the superficial soft-tissue envelope, defined by the platysma and structures superficial to this muscle (**Fig. 2**). Aging changes also occur in the deeper structural layers of the neck, including the subplatysmal fat, digastric muscles, and submandibular glands (**Fig. 3**). Because these deeper neck structures can be accessed through most rhytidectomy techniques, it is the authors' considered opinion that the most effective rhytidectomy

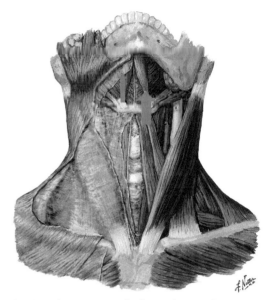

Fig. 2. Relevant centrally located muscular components for deep-plane neck lifting. The thin arrow points to the edge of the platysma muscle, which is deep to subcutaneous fat and part of the superficial cervical fascia. The thicker arrow points to the inferior end of the anterior belly of the digastric muscle, which is deep to the investing layer of the deep cervical fascia. Note that the digastric is deeper and more laterally based then the platysma muscle. (Netter illustration *from* www.netterimages. © Elsevier Inc. All rights reserved.)

approach to the neck is the technique that maximizes the surgeon's ability to mobilize and resuspend the entire superficial soft-tissue envelope.

Mitz and Peyronie[3] defined the superficial cervical facial fascia in 1976, demonstrating the SMAS

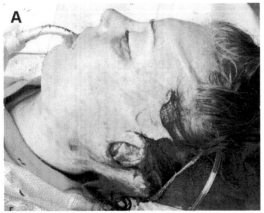
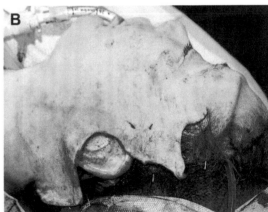

Fig. 1. Intraoperative photos demonstrating the excessive soft-tissue redundancy created after deep-plane dissection and mobilization of the facial soft tissues, even in the younger patient. This redundancy supports gravity's effects on facial soft tissue as the etiology in facial aging. Note the need to use hairline incisions to avoid the extreme superior displacement of the temporal hair tuft in these cases. (*A*) A 43-year-old woman undergoing deep plane face lift. (*B*) 59-year-old woman undergoing deep plane face lift.

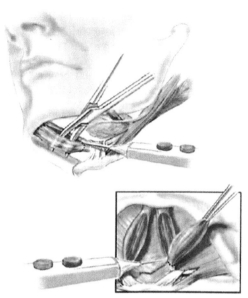

Fig. 3. The subplatysmal fat, digastric muscles, and submandibular glands are the central components of the deeper structural neck layers involved in the aging process. The procedure shown addresses the ptotic anterior digastric muscles by subtotal inferior excision. (*From* Connell BF. Contemporary concepts for correction of neck contour deformities. In: Eisenmann-Klein M, Neuhann-Lorenz C, editors. Innovations in plastic and aesthetic surgery. Berlin (Germany): Springer-Verlag; 2008. p. 225; with permission.)

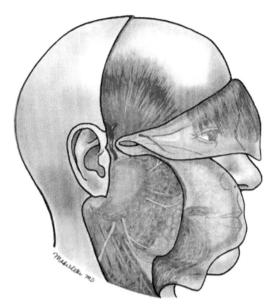

Fig. 4. Deep plane of the face is the embryologic cleavage plane separating the superficial soft-tissue envelope from the deeper structural aspects of the face that are bounded by the deep cervical fascia. (*Adapted from* Zoumalan RA, Larrabee WF. Anatomic considerations in the aging face. Facial Plast Surg 2011;27(1):18; with permission.)

to be a fibromuscular extension of the platysma muscle. Skoog[4] advanced facelift techniques by defining the significance of the sub-SMAS dissection. Further improvement was made by Hamra[5] in 1990 with his description of deep-plane rhytidectomy.

The deep plane of the face is defined as the embryologic cleavage plane separating the superficial soft-tissue envelope from the deeper structural aspects of the face, which are bounded by the deep cervical fascia (**Figs. 4** and **5**). Dissection of the midface in the sub-SMAS/deep plane creates multiple advantages that allow for significantly improved outcomes in face and neck lifting. First, this approach enables direct deep lysis of the zygomatic cutaneous ligament, which is the major facial retaining ligament[6]; direct assessment and treatment of issues such as pseudoherniation of buccal fat and its influence on jowling; and mobilization of most of the facial fat.[7] Second, because the SMAS is contiguous with the platysma muscle in the neck, sub-SMAS mobilization of the midface and superiorly/laterally based resuspension of the SMAS/platysma unit provide the best opportunity for significant and long-lasting neck rejuvenation.

Third, because the deep-plane flap resuspension confines tension to the platysma/SMAS fascia, the technique is preferable for revision rhytidectomy procedures whereby avoiding or reversing skin tension is paramount to the procedure's success. This concept further supports the deep-plane approach in treating "neck failures," which are often due to undercorrected vertical suspension of the SMAS/platysma unit in the midface

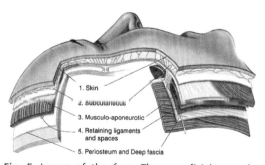

1. Skin
2. Subcutaneous
3. Musculo-aponeurotic
4. Retaining ligaments and spaces
5. Periosteum and Deep fascia

Fig. 5. Layers of the face. The superficial muscular aponeurotic system (SMAS) is the deep layer of the superficial soft tissue containing most of the facial fat distributed homogeneously superficial to the SMAS. (*Adapted from* Mendelson BC, Jacobson SR. Surgical anatomy of the midcheek: facial layers, spaces, and midcheek segments. Clin Plast Surg 2008;35(3):398; with permission.)

(Fig. 6).[8] Lastly, confined tension to the platysma/SMAS fascia allows for a tension-free skin closure, minimizes complications and results in a truly natural rejuvenation.

ANATOMY

By understanding the relevant facial anatomy and embryology, preference for the deep-plane rhytidectomy technique and its safe performance becomes evident. Initially viewing the layers of the face (see **Fig. 5**), one sees that the SMAS is the deep portion of the superficial soft-tissue envelope, with most facial fat distributed homogeneously superficial to this layer.[9] This embryologic boundary is contiguous from the platysma in the neck to the galea in the forehead (see **Fig. 4**).

Below this layer is the superficial layer of the deep cervical fascia, covering all the deeper embryologic structures such as the masseter muscle, facial nerve, and buccal fat pad (**Fig. 7**). The potential space located between these layers represents the embryologic cleavage plane of the midface that defines the deep plane. Dissection in this potential space in the midface is relatively avascular, and the facial nerve is securely protected by the deep cervical fascia. In addition, the SMAS fascia fuses with the superficial layer of the deep cervical fascia at the parotid gland and is poorly defined superiorly over the facial mimetic muscles, such as the zygomatic and orbicularis muscles. Thus, most of the malar fat pad sits on this superior group of facial mimetic muscles. Crossing through these planes are the 2 facial ligaments: at the body

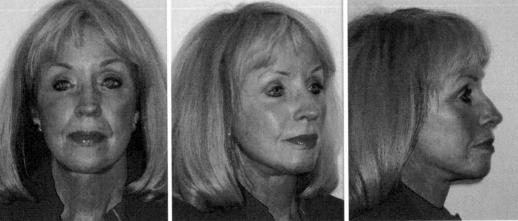

Fig. 6. Preoperative (A) and postoperative (B) photos of a 67-year-old woman treated with a revision deep-plane rhytidectomy, browlift, upper and lower blepharoplasty, and periocular and perioral Er:YAG laser skin resurfacing. The deep-plane facelift is the optimal approach for revision cases because tension is isolated on the fascia, preventing any further skin tension that would compromise natural results.

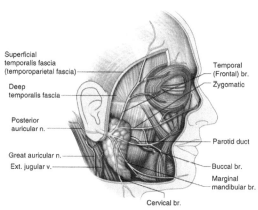

Superficial temporalis fascia (temporoparietal fascia)

Deep temporalis fascia

Posterior auricular n.

Great auricular n.

Ext. jugular v.

Temporal (Frontal) br.

Zygomatic

Parotid duct

Buccal br.

Marginal mandibular br.

Cervical br.

Fig. 7. Illustration of the facial anatomy in the deep plane. The superficial layer of the deep cervical fascia covers the deeper structures of the face such as the masseter muscle, facial nerve, and buccal fat. (*From* Tan KS, Oh SR, Priel A, et al. Surgical anatomy of the forehead, eyelids, and midface for the aesthetic surgeon. In: Massry GG, Murphy MR, Azizzadeh B, editors. Master techniques in blepharoplasty and periorbital rejuvenation. New York: Springer; 2011. p. 22; with permission.)

of the zygoma are the zygomatic cutaneous ligaments (McGregor patch) and inferiorly on the medial aspect of the mandible are the mandibular ligaments, which are the sole anchors of the facial soft-tissue envelope (**Fig. 8**).[6]

The deep plane is very well defined inferiorly along the masseter muscle because of the presence of platysma muscle in the SMAS fascia.

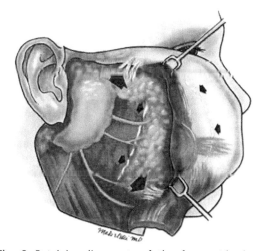

Fig. 8. Retaining ligaments of the face, with the SMAS elevated. Both the zygomatic ligament (McGregor patch) superiorly, and the mandibular ligament inferiorly, are strong ligaments with periosteal attachments (*wide arrows*). (*Adapted from* Zoumalan RA, Larrabee WF. Anatomic considerations in the aging face. Facial Plast Surg 2011;27(1):20; with permission.)

Superiorly, the deep plane is more poorly defined, as the fascia thins out at the level of the facial mimetic muscles. Continuing inferiorly, the midface is separated from the neck by the mandibular septum of the mandible, whose medial border is the mandibular ligament. The platysma is fully developed, continuing inferiorly as a muscular sheet in the neck with varying amounts of preplatysmal fat throughout this layer. Deeper structures include subplatysmal fat, the anterior bellies of the digastric muscle, and the submandibular glands that comprise the subplatysmal pertinent structures in neck rejuvenation, which are all centrally located (see **Fig. 3**).

EVALUATION

Evaluation of a surgical candidate should include standard medical clearance for a patient undergoing general anesthesia. The authors prefer that the patient be intubated under a propofol-based anesthetic. Often, facelift procedures are combined with browlifts and eyelid procedures. Physical evaluation should be based on the specific combination of procedures to be performed. The presence and degree of aging changes (such as the nasolabial folds, jowling, platysma banding, ptotic digastric/submandibular triangles, submental fat deposition and festoons) should be defined before the deep-plane facelift.[10,11] Normal anatomic variances, including facial dimples and the hyoid/mental relationship, are noted during the initial evaluation.[12]

From the perspective of the facial plastic surgeon, the importance of defining face type by palpation of the facial soft tissue cannot be overemphasized. Compliant faces will often manifest the effects of gravity at an earlier stage and create more soft tissue mobilization, thus requiring careful hairline planning. Stiff, noncompliant faces can be more difficult to dissect, but these typically will maintain their outcomes for a longer period of time. Thicker soft tissue will require more lateral/periauricular soft-tissue contouring when the flap is mobilized. The deep plane will be more proximal to the subcutaneous plane in thin faces.

Differentiating between superficial soft-tissue (from platysma to skin) and subplatysmal age-related changes is vital to produce optimal, predictable neck outcomes. The significance is revealed when optimal surgical treatment of the platysma unit is achieved in a patient with untreated subplatysmal age-related changes. The better the result in the superficial soft-tissue layer, the more accentuated the subplatysmal age-related changes may become after rhytidectomy. When viewing the neck the platysma component is typically medial, often continuing below the hyoid bone in the aging neck. The ptotic or thickened anterior digastric muscles (and/or ptotic submandibular glands) are more laterally located and are confined superior to the lateral aspect of the hyoid bone (see **Fig. 2**). Asking the patient to flex the platysma muscle can be helpful in defining which neck components are most prominent preoperatively. This examination may be very difficult in the severely aged or fatty neck, in which case anatomic landmarks become obscured (**Fig. 9**). In the majority of cases, most changes in the aging neck are confined to the superficial soft-tissue envelope.

Complete neurologic examination should document both trigeminal nerve status and facial nerve function. Photographs should document both static and dynamic images in frontal, three-quarter, and lateral views. Ear position and shape, facial asymmetries, and hairlines should be documented. Dynamic images should document patterns of muscle action.

PATIENT PERSPECTIVE

Patients desire a maximal aesthetic outcome with the least extensive process possible. The career and social demands of many patients require them to be cosmetically presentable in public within 2 weeks. An individual's aesthetic goals should be balanced with the stage of aging, and any anatomic limitations, such as festoons or ptotic digastric/submandibular triangles, should be discussed so that appropriate patient expectations and the best treatment plan can be defined. Risks and benefits should be discussed before any contemplated procedure. Minimally invasive procedures and their limitations should be presented as alternatives. "Before and after" photographs of the contemplated procedure with similarly profiled previous patients are helpful in establishing realistic expectations of outcomes.

THE DEEP-PLANE APPROACH TO NECK REJUVENATION
Surgical Procedure

Detailed surgical planning is crucial in aesthetic surgery. Intraoperative access to preoperative photographs is also essential. Although most of the authors' deep-plane facelifts are combined with other procedures, only the facelift portion of the procedure is described here (Video 1).

Anesthesia

Preference is for the procedures to be done under a propofol-based general anesthetic. Bleeding is controlled throughout the procedure by a surgical-field injection of a 1:1 mix of 1% lidocaine with 1:100,000 epinephrine and 0.5% bupivacaine with 1:200,000 epinephrine, combined with hypotensive anesthesia. Perioperative antibiotics covering skin flora and one dose of intravenous steroids are given before incision. Except for a short-acting agent for anesthesia induction, muscle relaxants are not used.

Patient Preparation

Once the patient has been anesthetized, the hair is cut and the patient marked accordingly (**Fig. 10**).

A retrotragal incision is typically used in women because the deep-plane procedure avoids tension on the incision lines, maintaining normal ear and tragal architecture. Pretragal incisions are necessary in men to avoid moving hair-bearing skin on to the tragus.

Because there is a significant degree of soft-tissue mobilization using the deep-plane technique, even in younger patients, the authors prefer to use temporal hairline incisions to avoid superior and posterior movement of the temporal hair tuft (see **Fig. 1**).

Based on the prediction of soft-tissue mobilization, the postauricular limb is designed more superiorly, with a more acute angle (compared with the antihelix), for patients with relatively compliant soft tissue. For patients with less compliant soft tissue or with revision cases, the postauricular limb is based more inferiorly with a more obtuse angle. When a significant degree of soft tissue is mobilized in the midface and neck, there is a greater need to extend incisions for accommodation of redundant soft tissue and avoidance of dog ears or tissue bunching.

Initial Incisions

Incisions are made using a #10 blade, ensuring to bevel at exposed hairlines for preservation of hair follicles, such as the anterior temporal tuft. Care is made to incise the skin at the edge of the tragus to hide the incision, thus avoiding the unnatural skin drape that would occur on closing an incision placed too far retrotragally. Cautery is not used at bleeding hairlines to preserve hair follicles. Application of a cold lap pad or sponge will often tamponade hairline bleeding.

It must be noted that with more significant soft-tissue mobilization there is greater need for extended incisions, both temporally and postauricularly. If a limited incision pattern is desired (such as eliminating the postauricular incision component), more limited deep-plane dissections can be done in concert with limited flap

A

B

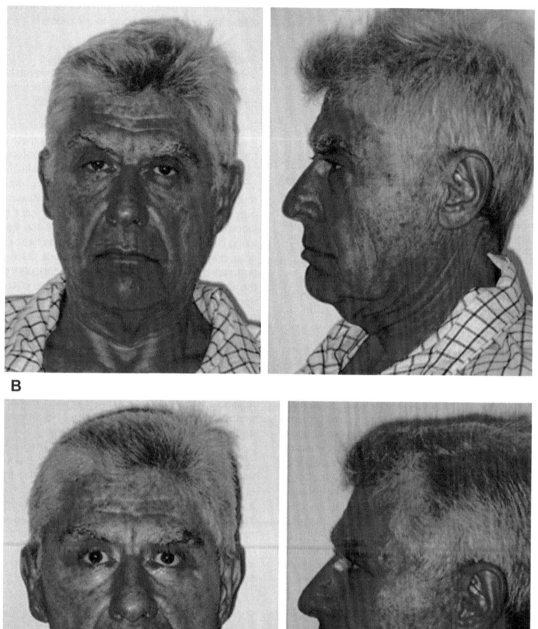

Fig. 9. Preoperative (*A*) and postoperative (*B*) photos of a 65-year-old man with severe neck changes. The subplatysmal aspects of neck aging are obscured in the advanced-aged neck. Treatment comprised deep-plane facelift, browlift, upper and lower blepharoplasty, and periocular Er:YAG laser skin resurfacing.

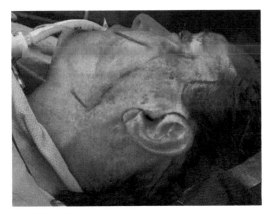

Fig. 10. Intraoperative photo showing marked hairline incision for maximal preservation of hairline. In addition, the diagonal line from angle of the mandible to lateral canthus demonstrates surface landmark of where the deep plane will be entered.

advancement and fixation. Care in planning is necessary to avoid bunching of soft tissue. Limited incision patterns also place constraints on the overall outcome.

Midface Dissection

Subcutaneous plane dissection
Sharp dissection then proceeds in the preauricular subcutaneous plane and is extended postauricularly. Dissection should be accomplished proximal to the facial musculature, with careful avoidance of the postauricular muscle and the great auricular nerve. Dissection is carried into the preplatysmal plane in the neck toward the midline. An effort is made to maximize the neck dissection from this approach. Sharp dissection is carried to the diagonal line extending from the angle of the mandible to the lateral border of the orbicularis oculi muscle (see **Fig. 10**). The angle of the mandible is used as a reference because it often represents the anterior border of the parotid gland. Because the

SMAS and the deep cervical fascia are fused on the parotid, the deep plane cannot be entered until dissection proceeds anterior to the parotid.

Deep-plane dissection
Safe entry into the deep plane can be achieved by creating reference points and using them when defining less obvious aspects of dissection.

First reference point: lateral border of orbicularis muscle The first reference point is established at the lateral border of the orbicularis muscle, inferior to the lateral canthus. In the deep plane, unlike the composite rhytidectomy, the orbicularis oculi muscle is not part of the flap (**Fig. 11**).[13,14] Maximal outcomes will best be achieved by taking care to incorporate most of the soft tissue into the flap along the superior facial mimetic muscles. Of note, some of the temporal-to-orbicularis dissection can be done bluntly; the ease of this part of the dissection often foreshadows the ease of the upcoming sub-SMAS dissection.

The deep plane is entered using a #10 blade to create a sharp edge, or shelf, which will be used to mobilize and fixate the complex flap at a later stage in the procedure.

Definition of the deep plane should first be accomplished just superior to the angle of the mandible, where masseter muscle is an obvious deep boundary and the SMAS is well developed and incorporated with platysma muscle.

Categorizing the patient's face type is integral to predicting plane depth. Thin faces tend to have a thin, poorly developed SMAS/platysma, and the difference between the subcutaneous dissection and the deep plane may be of minimal depth. The platysma muscle will first be encountered as the depth of dissection increases. Platysma can be recognized by its transverse muscle fibers, in contrast to the vertically oriented muscle fibers of the deeper masseter muscle.

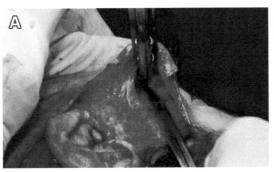
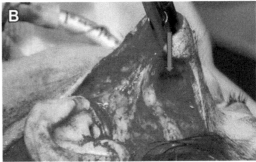

Fig. 11. (A, B) Intraoperative photos exhibiting the initial anatomic landmark used to define the deep-plane, orbicularis oculi muscle. Unlike the composite rhytidectomy, the orbicularis muscle is not part of the flap. An (arrow) indicates flap being raised.

Once beneath the SMAS, fibroareolar tissue representing the potential space defining the deep plane becomes evident (**Fig. 12**). At this point, it is easy to bluntly dissect the fibroareolar tissue to further establish the deep plane. Often, blunt dissection can glide along anteriorly past the masseter muscle to the perioral area with little resistance.

Second reference point: masseter muscle The second reference point of the masseter muscle now becomes evident, covered by the superficial layer of the deep cervical fascia, which also protects the underlying facial nerve. This reference point, along with the lateral border of the already defined orbicularis oculi muscle, permits the deep plane to be developed anteriorly over the masseter muscle, and the buccal fat pad toward the mouth.

Deep-plane development is carried superiorly to the inferior border of the zygomatic major muscle. The deep plane is usually avascular except around the zygoma and submalar regions. Bleeding may occur from the facial or labial arteries if dissection is traumatic. Because branches of the facial nerve accompany these arteries, monopolar cautery should be avoided, and simple pressure and hypotensive anesthesia will typically tamponade any bleeding that may be encountered.

At this point in the procedure, the only region yet to be dissected is the bridge of soft tissue inferior to the initial orbicularis dissection and superior to the masseter dissection.

Sharp dissection is necessary in this area, where the zygomatic cutaneous ligaments will be encountered. Release of these ligaments fully mobilizes the midface, especially the malar fat pad, and positively influences the nasolabial folds (**Fig. 13**).[15,16] The ligaments cannot be lysed bluntly; failure to release them severely limits the extent of midface mobilization and hinders

treatment outcome. Using the defined inferior and superior plane, one can comfortably cut through the retaining ligaments. Blunt dissection can typically be used to continue anteriorly along the zygomatic major muscle. Care is taken during this part of the dissection to incorporate most of the malar fat pad soft tissue into the flap, leaving a skeletonized zygomatic major muscle.

Nasolabial folds and oral commissure A combination of blunt and sharp dissection is carried out anteriorly to the nasolabial fold. Gentle dissection is used on approach to the oral commissure to protect the labial branch of the facial nerve, which becomes superficial and can be injured by overly vigorous dissection.

Dimples Of note, prior documentation of dimples is predictive of the anatomy of the zygomatic major muscle. Because a classic midface dimple is caused by either a fascial band extending from the zygomatic major muscle (minor dimple) or a frank bifid zygomatic major muscle (major dimple), care must be taken to preserve this offshoot of the zygomatic major muscle as it travels to the dermis inferiorly.

Assessment of deep facial structures The midface has been degloved in the embryologic cleavage plane at this point in the procedure (**Fig. 14**). Now the deep facial structures contributing to aging, such as the buccal fat pad, can be individually assessed.

The buccal fat pad is covered by the superficial layer of the deep cervical fascia. As the facial skeleton subtly shrinks, the fascia can become weak or ptotic, and cause the buccal fat pad to pseudoherniate. This process is similar to the concept of orbital fat pseudoherniation that contributes to ocular aging changes. The pseudoherniation of

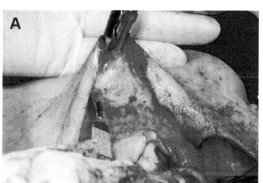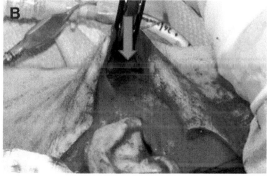

Fig. 12. (*A, B*) Intraoperative photos showing the establishment of the deep plane, just superior to the angle of the mandible. This anatomic landmark is used because the deep plane has a well-defined deep boundary, the masseter muscle, and a well-developed SMAS/platysma muscle unit. Fibroareolar tissue defines this potential space (*arrow*).

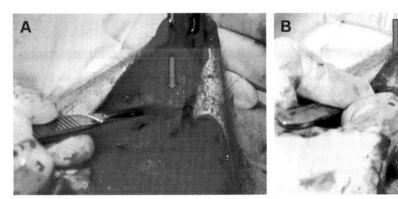

Fig. 13. (*A*, *B*) Intraoperative photos revealing sharp lysis of the zygomatic cutaneous ligament (*arrow*), which will allow malar fat pad repositioning for treatment of the nasolabial folds and restore facial width.

the buccal fat pad has the potential to contribute to jowling or even a "cheeky" appearance (**Fig. 15**), and can be individually assessed in vivo from the deep-plane dissection.

Because the patient is supine intraoperatively, a fullness or bulge of the buccal fat pad will understate its contribution to a jowl, and should be correlated with preoperative photos to make a precise judgment regarding the amount and position of buccal fat excision (**Fig. 16**).

If buccal fat pseudoherniation is present, the authors conservatively make a small nick incision through the fascia using sharp scissors. The surgical assistant applies pressure on the buccal fat pad, while a conservative amount of buccal fat is gently teased through the nick incision and resected using bipolar cautery, with strict observation for any facial twitches (**Fig. 17**). The contour change of the buccal fat pad immediately becomes more linear, often after excision of only a small amount of buccal fat. If too much buccal fat herniates through the nick incision, it should

be gently placed back into the subfascial pocket. This last maneuver completes the midface dissection, which is repeated on the contralateral side.

Neck Dissection

Incision

To complete the neck dissection, a horizontal submental incision is made either in the crease or slightly inferior, depending on submental anatomy. Preoperative photos are referenced to define the pattern, symmetry, and degree of platysma banding, fat deposition pattern, and contour of the submandibular/digastric triangle. Often the digastric muscle can be identified by following the muscle outlines extending to the lateral aspect of the hyoid bone, which then redirect posterior/superior. The platysma is differentiated by its more medial location, crossing and even obscuring the hyoid. The digastric-platysma distinction is important in guiding further neck treatment (see **Fig. 2**).

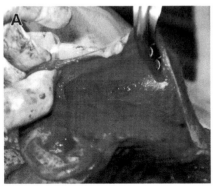
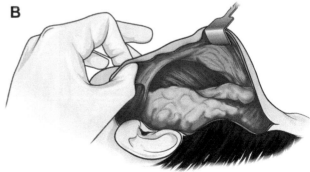

Fig. 14. (*A*) Intraoperative photo displaying a fully degloved midface in the deep plane. Retractor is tenting the zygomatic major muscle into view. A clear SMAS/platysma shelf is evident along the deep aspect of the flap. (*B*) A deep-plane dissection schematically representing similar structures.

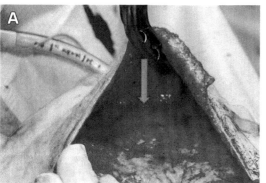
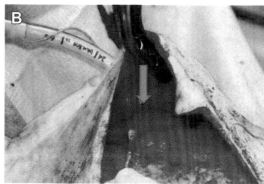

Fig. 15. (*A*, *B*) Intraoperative photos illustrating pseudoherniation of buccal fat pad in the supine position after deep-plane dissection (*arrow*). Note that the supine position minimizes the appearance of buccal fat pseudoherniation.

Preplatysmal and subplatysmal dissection and assessment

After incision, subsequent preplatysmal dissection will connect the submental dissection to the completed bilateral facial dissections. Care is taken to grasp only the redundant platysma muscle in the midline. After cross-clamping, redundant muscle is resected.

The next steps taken will be defined by the assessment of the contribution to aging of subplatysmal fat and digastric/submandibular gland in each case. Even when present, subplatysmal

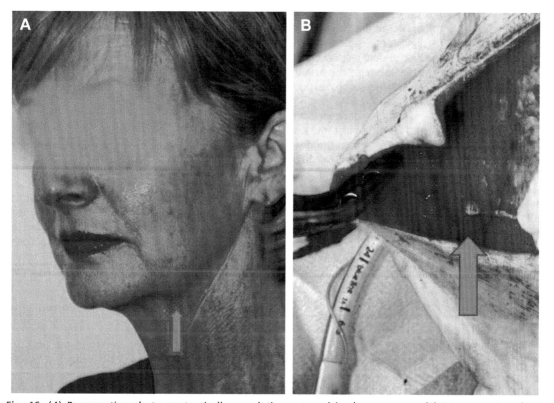

Fig. 16. (*A*) Preoperative photo anatomically correlating external jowl appearance. (*B*) Intraoperative photo revealing buccal fat pseudoherniation in same position, in the same patient (*arrow*). This view confirms the contribution of pseudoherniated buccal fat to jowling.

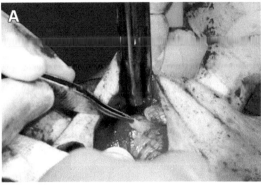
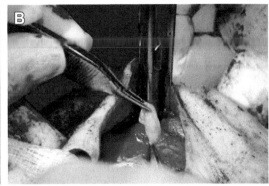

Fig. 17. (*A, B*) Intraoperative photos showing the technique for delivery of buccal fat. Mild pressure is applied to the buccal fat pad by the surgical assistant as a nick incision is made into the fascia, allowing precise removal of buccal fat.

aspects of neck aging are approached in a judicious, conservative fashion.

Dissection is carried out in the subplatysmal plane only until the anterior digastric muscle is exposed. Partial resection along the inferior aspect of the anterior digastric muscle is an option for the experienced surgeon (see **Fig. 3**).

Although it is well described, the authors do not resect submandibular glands because of associated increased risk to the marginal mandibular nerve.[17] Subplatysmal fat can be resected between the digastric muscles, although it is infrequently the most significant factor in fat deposition. This maneuver should especially be avoided when the digastric/submandibular triangle is ptotic because it can enhance and/or expose these aesthetic issues.

Often, a soft-tissue bulge between the mentum and the hyoid, not consistent with the ptotic platysma pattern, can signal the need for subplatysmal fat excision. Even in these cases, defatting should be approached conservatively to avoid a hollowing or "cobra deformity."

Platysma imbrication

Once subplatysmal fat excision is completed, the previously resected redundant platysma muscle is imbricated using buried Prolene sutures. 4-0 Prolene is often used proximal to the mentum, while 3-0 Prolene sutures are otherwise used until the hyoid bone is encountered.

Imbrication of the platysma should not proceed below the hyoid, to prevent bowstringing of the muscle. One small finger should fit in the gap between the muscle edge and the hyoid at completion of the imbrication. Even severely ptotic neck contours may not require significant platysma muscle resection.

Once the platysma muscle sling is created, preplatysmal fat contouring completes the neck component of the deep-plane rhytidectomy. Most fat contouring is done by sharp, direct dissection in the preplatysmal plane. Care is taken to maintain an even layer of fat on the muscle flap, preventing both irregularities and dermal-platysma adherence.

Completion of neck-contouring process

Completion of the entire neck-contouring process is confirmed by manually lifting the midface and viewing the recreated neckline. (This maneuver recapitulates the significance of vertically suspending the platysma/SMAS in the midface as the majority factor in improving the neck contour.) This action will reveal any contour irregularities that need addressing further. If an incomplete neck contour is evident, all components of neck aging should be reassessed to guide further treatment.

Once preplatysmal fat contouring is complete, the neck is copiously irrigated with multiple cool saline washes and one Betadine wash to minimize residual necrotic fat cells, which may serve as a future nidus of infection. Cautery is avoided on the skin flap to prevent delayed skin necrosis. The submental incision is closed with 5-0 Prolene sutures.

Flap Mobilization, Fixation, and Closure

Flap mobilization, fixation, and closure proceed. After initial hemostasis is achieved through use of bipolar cautery, a small bulb drain is placed through a postauricular hairline stab incision.

Because the thicker, deep-plane complex flap will be advanced and sutured proximate to the preauricular incision, case-specific preauricular soft-tissue contouring and resection is necessary.

The new depth created should be consistent with the thickness of the deep-plane flap that will be inlaid. This process ensures that the bulkiness of the complex flap does not create an aesthetic issue resulting in unnatural alterations of the normal preauricular and tragal architecture.

Subcutaneous contouring will also prevent facial widening from occurring. Subcutaneous tissue should only be resected to the parotid fascia, which must be kept intact for anchoring the advanced flap.

Depending on the degree of mobilization desired, the deep plane can also be extended inferiorly for a few centimeters below the angle of the mandible to incorporate more soft tissue into the advancement flap. This maneuver should be performed judiciously, with special care taken to avoid the marginal mandibular and platysmal branches of the facial nerve.

Hemostasis

In assessing the deep-plane dissection for bleeding before closure, bipolar cauterization of blood vessels should be cautiously minimized and the face monitored as necessary. Soft-tissue pressure and hypotensive anesthetic technique usually suffice for hemostasis.

Sutures

Flap advancement proceeds from inferior to superior using 3-0 Prolene sutures (**Fig. 18**). Commonly the SMAS fascia originating at the angle of the mandible can be advanced proximate to the earlobe. Subtle differences in the placement of the sutures will depend on variables such as flap thickness and soft-tissue compliance. Soft tissue is further contoured as necessary to recreate normal periauricular aesthetic architecture. The most superior suture of the advancement flap can be a 4-0 Prolene if the edge is thin.

Whereas maximal tension should be created at the level of the advancement flap fascia, minimal to no tension should be created at the skin level for the rest of the closure. A #11 blade is used to accurately tack the flap at the superior aspect of the helix as it connects to the temporal incision with 5-0 Prolene, used for the remainder of the skin closure.

The final extent of the anterior temporal skin incision is completed based on avoidance of soft-tissue bunching or formation of dog-ears. Meticulous soft-tissue tailoring using SuperCut scissors and a #15 blade provides sharp, crisp edges. Mattress sutures are used at the edge of hairlines.

Closure continues postauricularly in a similar fashion, using a tacking suture to match up the posterior hairline. The extent of the posterior incision is also completed inferiorly, again based on avoiding soft-tissue bunching or dog-ears. Precise soft-tissue tailoring is carried out to define the earlobe (using the preoperative photos as a reference) and to produce a tension-free preauricular skin closure. Maintenance of the tragal shape and other innate details are of utmost importance for creating subtle incision lines (**Fig. 19**).

Postprocedure

Once the procedure is completed, topical antibiotic ointment is applied to all incisions and a compression dressing is placed. If neck drains are present they are placed on bulb suction. Blood-pressure spikes are avoided during anesthesia emergence and extubation.

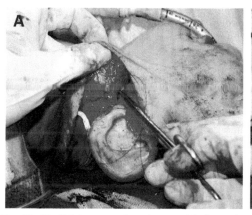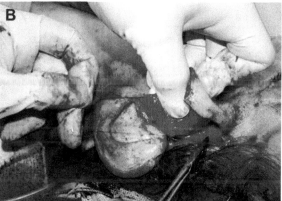

Fig. 18. (*A, B*) Intraoperative photos with flap advancement proceeding from inferior to superior using 3-0 Prolene sutures. The SMAS fascia originating at the angle of the mandible can be typically advanced proximate to the earlobe. Tension should be placed on this layer.

A

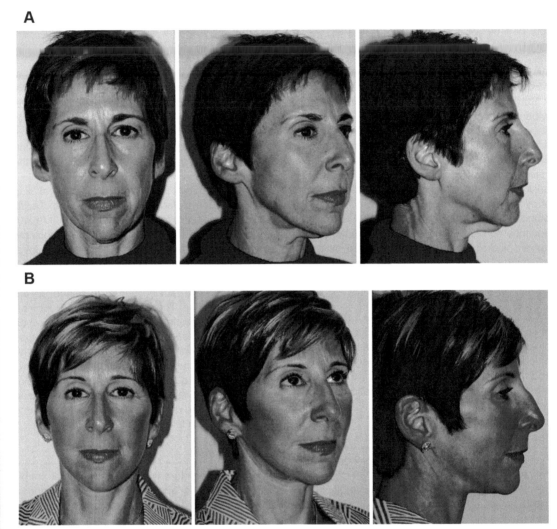

B

Fig. 19. Preoperative (*A*) and postoperative (*B*) photos of a 59-year-old woman with obvious platysma banding and minimal subplatysmal neck changes. She was treated with a deep-plane facelift, browlift, upper and lower blepharoplasty, and periocular Er:YAG laser skin resurfacing. Note the recreation of her facial shape at both the midface and jawline, and complete treatment of her platysma banding.

Aftercare

The compression dressing is removed on the morning of postoperative day 1. Often 2 small drains are used in the neck in deep-plane facelift procedures and are removed with the dressing. Incision lines are gently cleaned with hydrogen peroxide, and topical antibiotic ointment is applied 3 times daily. Visible sutures (such as those in the temporal hairline, submental, and preauricular regions) are removed on postoperative day 4. The remaining sutures are removed on postoperative day 7. Incision lines are sealed with colloidal and paper tape until they are subjectively defined as mature. Topical scar solution is then applied daily for 2 weeks. Activity is restricted for the first 2 weeks, with general guidelines given to keep the head elevated above the heart and to maintain heart rate and blood pressure within their relative normal ranges.

Complications

The complex flap created by the deep-plane dissection is well vascularized, and this makes it resistant to many rhytidectomy complications.[18,19] The rate of hematoma formation is reported to be as low as 1.8%, and is usually in the neck.[20,21] Infections are rare, reported at only 0.3% and 0.6% of cases, and are usually limited to the non–deep-plane areas such as the neck.[22] In 17 years, the authors have never seen an infection in the midface. Skin slough rates are also low, reported in

0% to 2.7% of cases, and are also limited to non–deep-plane portions of the dissection.[21,23] The advancement of the well-vascularized flap allows for deep-plane procedures to be performed safely in smokers.[20] The rate of facial nerve injury is 0.7%, similar to that of standard facelifts, and has not occurred in the authors' experience.[24]

SUMMARY

Most aging changes in neck contour are due to gravity's effects on the poorly anchored soft-tissue envelope, which creates excessive soft-tissue redundancy. Because access to neck structures is similar in most rhytidectomy procedures, the rhytidectomy technique that maximizes soft-tissue mobilization offers the best opportunity for recreating neck contour. Anatomic analysis of aging and embryologic evidence both support surgical facial degloving in the sub-SMAS plane and resuspension of the platysma/SMAS unit as the optimal surgical approach for mobilizing most of the ptotic facial soft tissue. Vertical resuspension of the platysma/SMAS complex not only

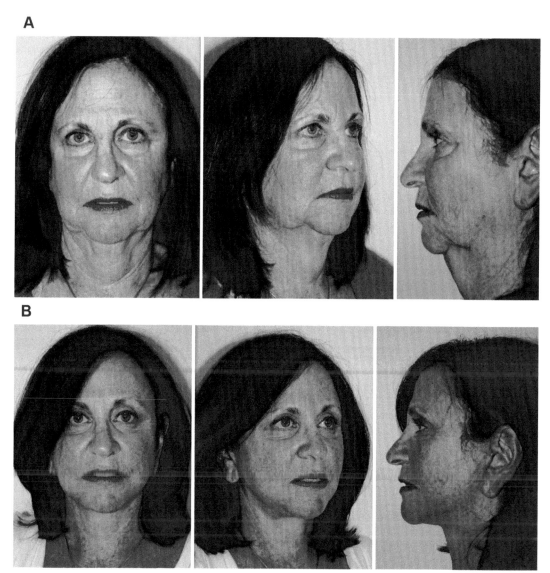

A

B

Fig. 20. Preoperative (A) and postoperative (B) photos of a 59-year-old woman with severe aging changes obscuring preoperative distinction between preplatysmal and subplatysmal neck abnormality. She was treated with a deep-plane facelift, browlift, upper and lower blepharoplasty, and periocular and perioral Er:YAG laser skin resurfacing. Note the improvement in facial shape, jowling, and neck contour, without hairline displacement or signs of surface tension, in a patient with a heavy face and significant aging changes.

best reproduces the midfacial contour but also accounts for most of the recreated neck and jawline (see **Figs. 18–20).**

The well-vascularized deep-plane flap minimizes complications. Outcomes can be maximized because tension exists "invisibly," only at the fascia level. This technique maximizes the surgeon's abilities in primary rhytidectomy procedures, and is preferred in revision procedures during which "neck failures" are often due to inadequately suspended SMAS/platysma in the midface (see **Fig. 6).** Overall significant, natural, and long-lasting aesthetic results are consistently achieved.

SUPPLEMENTARY DATA

Supplementary data related to this article can be found at http://dx.doi.org/10.1016/j.fsc.2014.01. 003.

REFERENCES

1. Ellenbogen R, Karlin JV. Visual criteria for success in restoring the youthful neck. Plast Reconstr Surg 1980;66:826–37.
2. Shaw RB, Katzel EB, Koltz F, et al. Aging of the facial skeleton: aesthetic implications and rejuvenation strategies. Plast Reconstr Surg 2011;127(1):374–83.
3. Mitz V, Peyronie M. The superficial musculo-aponeurotic system (SMAS) in the parotid and cheek area. Plast Reconstr Surg 1976;58:80–8.
4. Skoog TG. Plastic surgery: the aging face. In: Skoog TG, editor. Plastic surgery: new methods and refinements. Philadelphia: Saunders; 1974. p. 300–30.
5. Hamra ST. The deep-plane rhytidectomy. Plast Reconstr Surg 1990;86:53.
6. Furnas DW. The retaining ligaments of the cheek. Plast Reconstr Surg 1989;83:11–6.
7. Raskin E, LaTrenta GS. Why do we age in our cheeks? Aesthet Surg J 2007;27:19–28.
8. Gordon NA. Revision rhytidectomy: technique, modifications, and indications. Presented at the 10th International Symposium on Facial Plastic Surgery & American Academy of Facial Plastic and Reconstructive Surgery. Hollywood (FL), April 29, 2010.
9. Rohrich RJ, Pessa JE. The fat compartments of the face: anatomy and clinical implications for cosmetic surgery. Plast Reconstr Surg 2007;119:2219–27 [discussion: 2228–31].
10. Barton FE Jr. Rhytidectomy and the nasolabial fold. Plast Reconstr Surg 1992;90:601.
11. Gordon NA, Rosenberg R. Deep plane rhytidectomy: technical modifications, nuances, and observations, a 17 year experience. Master's seminar AAFPRS annual meeting. Washington, DC, September 6, 2012.
12. Brennan HG, Kock RJ. Management of the aging neck. Facial Plast Surg 1996;12(3):241–55.
13. Hamra ST. Composite rhytidectomy. Plast Reconstr Surg 1992;90(1):1–13.
14. Hamra ST. Composite Rhytidectomy. St. Louis (MO): Quality Medical Publishing; 1993.
15. Yousif NJ, Gosain A, Matloub HS, et al. The nasolabial fold: an anatomic and histologic reappraisal. Plast Reconstr Surg 1994;93:60.
16. Owsley JQ. Lifting the malar fat pad for correction of prominent nasolabial folds. Plast Reconstr Surg 1993;91:4634.
17. de Pina DP, Quinta WC. Aesthetic resection of the submandibular salivary gland. Plast Reconstr Surg 1991;88:779–87.
18. Whetzel TP, Mathes SJ. The arterial blood supply of the face lift flap. Plast Reconstr Surg 1997;100: 480–6.
19. Schuster RH, Gamble WB, Hamra ST, et al. A comparison of flap vascular anatomy in three rhytidectomy techniques. Plast Reconstr Surg 1995;95(4):683–90.
20. Parikh S, Jacono A. Deep-plane face-lift as an alternative in the smoking patient. Arch Facial Plast Surg 2011;13(4):283–5.
21. Grover R, Jones BM, Waterhouse N. The prevention of haematoma following rhytidectomy: a review of 1078 consecutive facelifts. Br J Plast Surg 2001; 54(6):481–6.
22. Zoumalan R, Rosenberg D. Methicillin-resistant *Staphylococcus aureus*-positive surgical site infections in face-lift surgery. Arch Facial Plast Surg 2008;10(2):116–23.
23. Rees TD, Liverett DM, Guy CL. The effect of cigarette smoking on skin-flap survival in the face lift patient. Plast Reconstr Surg 1984;73(6): 911–5.
24. Gordon NA, Godin M, Johnson CM. The deep plane rhytidectomy: technique, modifications and outcome of three hundred cases. Presented at American Academy of Facial Plastic and Reconstructive Surgery Annual Meeting. Washington, DC, September 27, 1996.

Vertical Neck Lifting

Andrew A. Jacono, MD[a,b,c,d,*], Benjamin Talei, MD[d,e]

KEYWORDS

- Vertical neck lift • Facelift • Rhytidectomy • Deep plane facelift • Platysmaplasty • SMAS
- Vertical facelift • Zygomatic cutaneous ligaments

KEY POINTS

- The authors' vertical neck lifting procedure is an extended deep plane facelift, which elevates the skin and superficial muscular aponeurotic system (SMAS)-platysma complex as a composite unit.
- The goal is to redrape cervicomental laxity vertically onto the face rather than laterally and postauricularly.
- The authors consider this an extended technique because it lengthens the deep plane flap from the angle of the mandible into the neck to release the cervical retaining ligaments that limit platysmal redraping.
- This technique does not routinely use midline platysmal surgery because it counteracts the extent of vertical redraping.
- A majority of aging face patients are good candidates for this procedure in isolation, but indications for combining vertical neck lifting with submental surgery are elucidated.

INTRODUCTION

Restoration of a youthful jawline and neck is an integral part of facial rejuvenation and arguably the most important goal for patients and doctors alike in aging face surgery. As the middle-aged population has grown and plastic surgery of the face has gained increasing acceptance, more patients are seeking cervicofacial rejuvenation at an earlier age; it is not uncommon to see patients in their 40s pursuing cervicofacial rhytidectomy. Even if the jowls are eliminated, residual neck redundancy may render the procedure a failure. The authors' practice has noted that undertreatment of the neck is probably the most common reason for patients to seek revision rhytidectomy within the first 3 years after a primary facelift.

Although aesthetic ideals may differ between various surgeons and patients, a majority aspire to recreate a neck and jawline similar to those described by Ellenbogen and Karlin.[1] Using a 26-year-old model, they establish 5 visual criteria believed to strike the eye as youthful after rhytidectomy: (1) distinct inferior mandibular border, (2) subhyoid depression, (3) visible thyroid cartilage bulge, (4) visible anterior sternocleidomastoid muscle (SCM) border, and (5) SM-SM angle of 90° (cervicomental angle between 105° and 120°).

Approaches to Achieve Aesthetic Ideal

To attain these aesthetic ideals, there have been myriad surgical approaches to address the issues existing in the lamina of the neck (ie, the skin, subcutaneous fat, and platysma and subplatysmal spaces). Choosing among the many different options requires a through physical examination. Surgeons must define which layers require

[a] Facial Plastic and Reconstructive Surgery, North Shore University Hospital, Community Drive, Manhasset, NY 11030, USA; [b] Facial Plastic Surgery, The New York Eye and Ear Infirmary, E 14th Street, New York, NY 10009, USA; [c] Department of Otorhinolaryngology, Head and Neck Surgery, The Albert Einstein College of Medicine, Morris Park Ave, Bronx, NY 10461, USA; [d] Facial Plastic Surgery, The New York Center for Facial Plastic and Laser Surgery, 5th Avenue, New York, NY 10075, USA; [e] Facial Plastic Surgery, The Beverly Hills Center for Plastic and Laser Surgery, Beverly Hills, CA 90210, USA
* Corresponding author. Facial Plastic and Reconstructive Surgery, North Shore University Hospital, Manhasset, NY 11030.
E-mail address: drjacono@gmail.com

manipulation and identify neck habitus that leads to poor neck lift outcomes. These include excessive supraplatysmal fat, redundant platymsa with vertical banding, and excessive fat or submandibular gland ptosis in the subplatymsa space. Those with a low anterior hyoid have a blunted cervicomental angle resulting from low insertion of the anterior belly of the digastric and the floor of mouth musculature. These specific problems limit a surgeon's ability to redrape neck redundancy and create the 105° to 120° cervicomental angle.

Barring patients with these specific anatomic configurations, the 2 most essential layers to manipulate in neck lifting are the skin/subcutaneous tissues and the SMAS-platysma complex. Although advances in rhytidectomy techniques have drastically improved aesthetic outcomes, there is a lack of consensus as to the preferred approach to the neck. Since the description of the SMAS layer by Skoog in 1974,[2] investigators have described a large variety of modifications of the sub-SMAS rhytidectomy. In 1976, Mitz and Peyronie[3] described the 2-layer rhytidectomy.

Bidirectional Technique

Since 1976, several influential surgeons have independently adapted and modified the extent of SMAS dissection technique, including Connell,[4] Owsley,[5,6] Barton,[7] Baker and Stuzin.[8–11] All these surgeons use the bidirectional cervicofacial rhytidectomy developed by Owsley that pulls the skin and SMAS-platysma complex in different directions with different amounts of tension.[12] In his original description of this bidirectional technique, the SMAS-platysma complex is elevated in a more superior or vertical fashion, and the skin is delaminated and redraped in a more lateral fashion. The benefits of a more vertical vector for SMAS directional pull have been recognized in both limited[13,14] and extensive dissection techniques.[4,7–11,15,16] An additional submental incision and central platysmal plication[9,17] is the preferred approach for extensive aging neck changes. These techniques have produced reliable and consistent outcomes.

Bidirectional and Vertical Technique Compared

The authors' vertical neck lifting technique differs from the bidirectional technique in 2 ways. First, both the SMAS-platysma complex and the skin are redraped in a more vertical vector. Additionally, the authors' dissection involves release of the facial retaining ligaments as part of the dissection to allow for greater vertical elevation of the platysma, SMAS, and neck skin.

Proponents of lamellar dissection and bidirectional rhytidectomy contend that the skin and SMAS age at different rates and along different vectors,[16] implying that the SMAS descends along a vertical gravitational vector but the skin along a horizontal vector. Dynamic examination of the preoperative rhytidectomy candidate reveals a greater laxity of the skin in the vertical vector than the horizontal vector in both the neck and lower cheek alike. This indicates the majority of aging of the skin occurs in the gravitational or vertical plane.

Skin Redraping

On closer examination of the bidirectional technique, horizontal skin redraping is performed to minimize superior temporal hairline displacement and temporal skin bunching that is associated with more vertical skin shifting techniques.[12,16] Additionally, it limits the length of the temporal incision and hides more of the incision in the postauricular region as the skin redundancy is removed posteriorly. In vertical skin redraping techniques, temporal hairline shifts can be managed by appropriate modification of the anterior incision by using an extended pretemporal hair tuft incision. To avoid bunching, the temporal skin must be undermined subcutaneously and redraped. These techniques are discussed later.

There are other inherent problems with horizontal skin redraping that warrant re-evaluation of this approach. Horizontal skin redraping has a greater propensity to create a lateral sweep deformity along the lower face and mandible. Lateral tension on the skin creates a horizontal tension bar across the cheek from the perioral region extending laterally and superiorly toward the ear. In more severe cases, this has been described as a joker line cross-cheek depression from the oral commissure.[18] This problem of the lateral tension vector was also described by Hamra as a "lateral sweep deformity."[19] This problem can be fixed with a revision rhytidectomy that redrapes the skin and the SMAS-platysma complex in a vertical antigravitational vector (**Fig. 1**).

Another issue with more lateral redraping of the facelift skin flap is that it limits the degree of definition at the cervicomental angle, one of the primary goals of rhytidectomy espoused by Ellenbogen and Karlin.[1] When the facelift skin flap is redraped in a more lateral fashion, the neck skin is tightened against the anterior neck overlying the hyoid and thyroid cartilages. In those patients with more redundant neck skin, this movement results in less redraping of the skin anterior to the hyoid, creating submental bunching and paramedian cervical pleating (**Fig. 2**). Even though this may not be

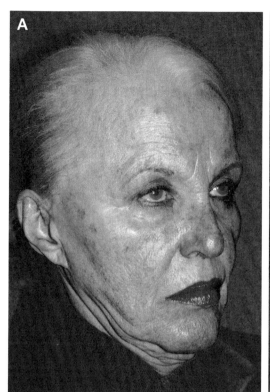 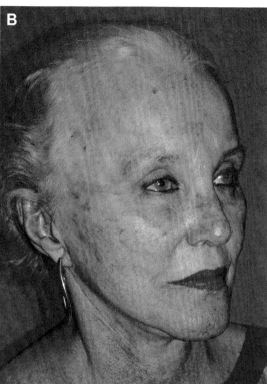

Fig. 1. (A) This 68-year-old woman was status post–prior rhytidectomy performed elsewhere 3 years earlier that resulted in a lateral sweep deformity and lateral facial pleating associated with horizontal skin redaping; (B) 12 months after vertical reorientation facelift to redrape the cheek skin in a vertical antigravitational vector. Because a deep plane technique was used, the skin and SMAS-platysma complex were redraped as 1 unit. Note the effacement of the lateral facial pleats.

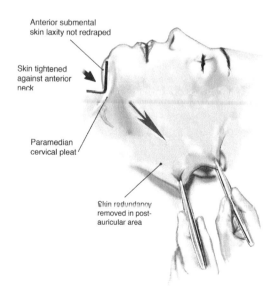

Anterior submental skin laxity not redraped

Skin tightened against anterior neck

Paramedian cervical pleat

Skin redundancy removed in post-auricular area

Fig. 2. With lateral neck skin redraping during rhytidectomy, skin is tightened against the anterior neck overlying the hyoid and thyroid cartilages, resulting in anterior submental bunching and paramedian cervical pleating.

evident in the early postoperative period, it may become evident as the skin relaxes over the first 6 to 12 months after surgery. This approach is favored by many surgeons because it places most of the rhytidectomy scar in the posterior auricular region. The authors noticed these anterior submental failures in their practice prior to adopting the vertical technique approximately 7 years ago. Increasing experience with this technique has led the authors to notice this issue more often in patients presenting for a revision neck lift consultation after primary surgery (Fig. 3).

Vertical elevation of the rhytidectomy flap maximizes redraping of the neck skin into the cervicomental angle, hence enhancing its definition. The minimal access cranial suspension (MACS) lift originally described by Tonnard and colleagues[20] pioneered a purely vertical elevation of the skin and SMAS to accomplish cervicomental rejuvenation and limit the posterior auricular scar. In the authors' technique, the skin flap is redraped more vertically, although not at a purely 90° angle with the horizontal, hence the term, *vertical neck lift*, is somewhat a misnomer. Purely vertical lifting

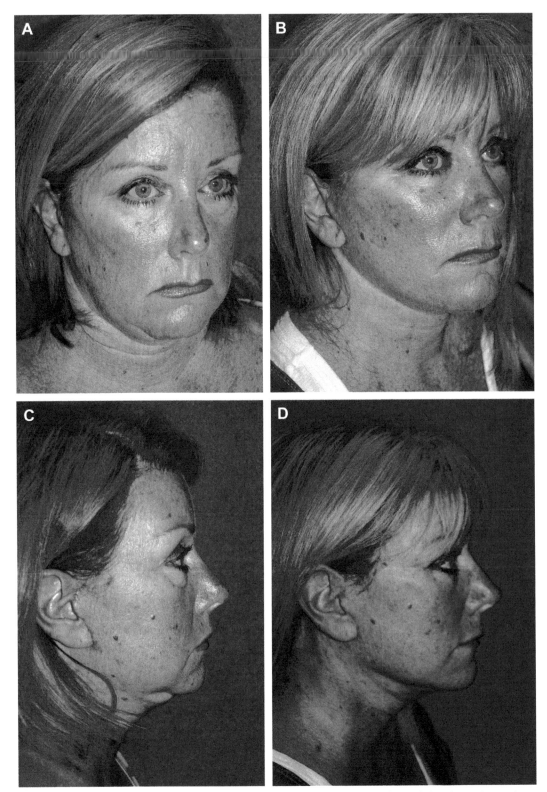

Fig. 3. (*A*, *C*) This 54-year-old woman was status post–biplanar rhytidectomy performed elsewhere 18 months previously with a lateral vector of neck skin redraping that resulted in anterior submental failure; (*B*, *D*) 12 months after vertical reorientation face and neck lift to redrape the neck skin in a vertical antigravitational vector into the cervicomental angle.

tightens the neck skin against the submentum overlying the floor of mouth musculature (digastric and mylohyoid region). It does not conform tightly into the cervicomental angle, resulting in anterior skin neck laxity.

The authors studied the angle of maximal redraping of the neck skin flap into the cervicomental angle. The facelift was performed as originally described by Hamra,[21] but with the modification of extending the deep plane below the angle of the mandible into the neck.[22,23] After complete elevation of the flap, the flap is placed under a moderate amount of tension and then rotated through a medially based arc. Rotation begins from directly horizontal (0°) and moves toward the vertical axis (90°); for the left hemiface, this is counterclockwise whereas the right is clockwise. The angle that results in the greatest reduction of submental laxity and jowling was calculated using vector calculations from the excised vertical and horizontal skin excess. The average angle of redraping required was 60°, creating maximal cervical rejuvenation. This indicates that the flap is redraped more vertically than a purely superolateral angle of 45°. With this vector of flap displacement, the majority of neck skin redundancy is shifted superiorly and is removed in the temporal region rather than in the postauricular region (**Fig. 4**). This effectively decreases the length of the posterior hairline incisions. The 60° angle is approximately parallel to a line drawn that bisects the cervicomental angle, tightening the redundant neck skin into this concavity.

SMAS-platysma Complex

As discussed previously, to counter the effects of aging and gravity, the authors prefer a more vertical vector of redraping for both the SMAS-platysma complex and the skin. With the deep plane technique, the SMAS-platysma complex is left connected to the skin in the majority of the facelift flap and thus lifted in the same direction. These vectors can similarly be accomplished using a biplanar technique by elevating the delaminated SMAS and skin independently in a more vertical vector. The 60° angle that contours the cervicomental region also approximately parallels the zygomaticus major muscle, which is the vector of pull placed on the SMAS in a bidirectional high SMAS facelift.[16]

Although the mean angle of redraping with the authors' technique is 60°, vectors calculated in this study ranged from 40° to the 70°s. The 3-D structure of the skeleton as well as the degree of laxity present dictate where the sweet spot or direction of maximal redraping of the soft tissue envelope exists in each face; it is not a cookie-cutter approach. A statistically significant inverse relationship is noted when comparing the angle of greatest redraping with age: older patients in their 70s develop greater horizontal laxity of their tissue nearing 40° whereas younger patients in their 40s have more vertical facial redundancy requiring a vector of pull approaching 70°.

The importance of vertical displacement of the SMAS-platysma complex in this technique must be emphasized. Because neck failure is the most common issue requiring tuck-up surgery after rhytidectomy, appropriate mobilization of the deeper layers is crucial, especially in those with platysmal banding and cording. To understand how this can be accomplished, further elucidation of the anatomy of the SMAS and platysma is necessary as is what limits the SMAS-platysma complex's motion.

The platysma has a higher extension onto the face than is classically illustrated in a variety of texts. A study of 71 consecutive deep plane rhytidectomies demonstrated that, on average, the platysma extends approximately 4 cm above the mandibular border into the cheek.[24] The significance of this should not be overlooked for several reasons. First, this suggests that the platysma plays a larger role than previously thought with regard to facial rejuvenation with use and manipulation of the SMAS-platysma complex. Most importantly, it suggests that redundancy of platysma in the neck has a significant contribution from inferior displacement of the platysma from the cheek. This anatomy elucidates that platysmal redraping should occur more superiorly than laterally as is traditionally performed. Fogli and Desouches[25] have promoted a technique that elevates the cervical portion of the platysma and

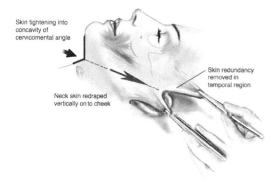

Skin tightening into concavity of cervicomental angle

Skin redundancy removed in temporal region

Neck skin redraped vertically on to cheek

Fig. 4. The most effective skin vector to tighten redundant neck skin into the cervicomental angle is approximately parallel to a line drawn that bisects the cervicomental angle. The authors' studies noted this angle is on average 60° with the horizontal, which is also parallel to the arc of the zygomaticus musculature.

anchors it to the malar periosteum, parotid fascia, and prelobar fibrous tissue. Cadaver studies comparing superolateral and vertical lifting of the SMAS-platysma complex further emphasize the importance of the vertical vector. Following intervention, Superolateral lifting was found to increase midline platysma dehiscence whereas it actually decreased after a vertical lift.[26]

The SMAS-platysma complex can be mobilized with suture techniques, such as lateral platysma plication sutures or platysmal flap elevation. Even with subplatysmal dissection and release, there are tethering points and retaining ligaments that limit motion of the deeper tissues. These fibers, described as the retinacular cutis, are located in relatively constant spaces and connect dermis down through the subcutaneous tissues, SMAS, and the muscle and periosteum overlying the facial skeleton.[27–30] They create anchoring points and septations between fat compartments that restrict redraping of the facial tissues. The importance of these retaining ligaments with regard to structure, shadowing, surgical implications,[28–33] and relation to the facial nerve[27–31,34–41] has been meticulously outlined.[27,28,42–45] Theoretically and conceptually, these zones serve as fulcra around which the pendular descent of soft tissues and skin occurs with aging and gravity.

Ligament Release

The important fibrous attachments to release in a vertical neck lift are the cervical retaining ligaments, the zygomatic cutaneous ligament,[46] and the mandibular cutaneous ligament (Fig. 5).[47,48] Retaining ligaments exist in the neck that anchor the platysma to the deep fascia of the overlying the SCM, significantly limiting the mobility of the platysma.[17] Limited subplatysmal dissection restricts the degree of neck mobilization and limits the extent of cervical rejuvenation. Releasing the cervical retaining ligaments allows for more significant redraping of the platysmal and midline cervical banding. Cadaver studies have been performed by the senior author (AAJ) comparing suture elevation of the platysma with release of the SMAS-platysma complex in a deep plane dissection extending into the neck. The deep plane dissection in this study included release of the cervical retaining ligaments. This study demonstrated there was a 554% greater redraping of submental platysmal laxity with the extended deep plane technique compared with SMAS-platysmal plication.[47] There are several important clinical implications of these data. First, retaining ligament release has the advantage of minimizing the need for midline platysmal plication. The senior author has demonstrated this in a cohort of 323 patients, where using a greater lateral platysmal release with deep plane surgery reduced the rate of platysmal plication to 13%.[49] Other investigators have claimed that they have completely eliminated the need for midline platysmoplasty with greater lateral release of the platysma[48] but it is the authors' experience that banding and redundancy associated with more advanced aged necks require midline platysmal reduction and plication combined with lateral platysmal release and elevation.

Midline plication

Limiting midline platysmal plication has further benefits in the vertical neck lift. Midline platysmal tightening directly counteracts the superior lifting of the neck tissues, thereby limiting the degree of potential improvement in the neck and jawline (Fig. 6). Siwani and Friedman[26] quantified this in

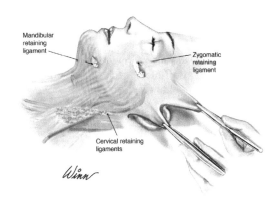

Fig. 5. The cervical retaining ligaments of the platysma, the zygomatic cutaneous ligament, and the mandibular cutaneous ligament limit vertical motion of the SMAS-platysma complex and neck skin in rhytidectomy.

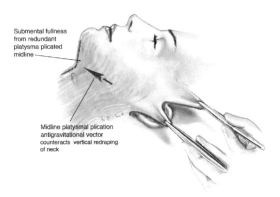

Fig. 6. Midline platysmal tightening directly counteracts the superior lifting of the neck tissues, thereby limiting the degree of improvement in the neck and jawline. Midline platysma binding also pulls the redundant platysma into the suprahyoid submentum adding bulk.

their cadaveric dissections, showing that the addition of platysma plication in facelift reduced the amount of total lift at points along the jawline by approximately 40%. Further disadvantages of midline approaches include an additional incision, increased operative time, and increased recovery time and, most importantly, fullness and irregularities in the submentum. Midline platysma binding pulls the redundant platysma into the suprahyoid submentum, adding bulk, and potentially creates postsurgical irregularities that are difficult to correct. Adding bulk to this region also minimizes the desired definition of the neck in the cervicomental angle around the hyoid, as described by Ellenbogen.[1]

Zygomatic-cutaneous ligaments

The zygomatic-cutaneous ligaments penetrate the upper border of the SMAS and bind it solidly to the zygoma.[28,30,35,41] Their release is necessary to allow for vertical elevation of the SMAS-platysma complex from the neck to the inferior cheek (along the jawline) and into the upper cheek where the ligaments reside. Biomechanical studies have shown the zygomatic ligaments not only are the strongest ligament of the face but also have the least elongation or stretch.[50] Because of how tightly they tether the skin, their release is also required to prevent bunching in the periorbital region when redraping redundant skin from the neck vertically into the midface and removing it in the temporal region. The necessity of ligamentous release to limit bunching and improve drapage was originally described by McGregor in the 1950s.[46]

Mandibular cutaneous ligaments

The mandibular cutaneous ligaments, although often overlooked, can have significant implications in neck lifting surgery. The mandibular ligament is an osteocutaneous ligament that arises from the anterior third of the mandible and inserts directly into the dermis.[27,28,30,33] Langevin and colleagues[51] reported the dimensions of the ligament measuring 2 cm horizontally and 1.2 cm vertically, positioned 4.5 cm anterior to the angle of the mandible.[51] The clinical importance of this ligamentous complex in rhytidectomy surgery was originally described by Furnas,[28] who noted that their release was required to adequately redrape the prejowl sulcus that is anterior to the jowl. He further noted that the cutaneous extension of this ligament causes skin indentations that can be magnified after rhytidectomy, ultimately causing patient dissatisfaction.[28]

In vertical neck lifting, the authors have noted that the mandibular ligaments can also limit submental rejuvenation. The senior author has been measuring the clinical skin tethering effect of the mandibular ligament along the mandibular margin in 75 consecutive patients. This ligament limits motion of the skin along the jawline on average 5 cm posterior to the symphysis (Andrew A. Jacono, MD, personal communications, 2013). This tethering limits mobilization and redraping of the submental skin directly inferior and anterior to the mandibular ligament as it is lifted vertically. This results in anterior submental redundancy and recurrent neck ptosis in the early postoperative period (**Fig. 7**). When this occurs, a secondary procedure is often required, such as tuck-up neck lift surgery or a variety of other direct neck excision procedures. These sequelae are more problematic in necks with greater skin redundancy. As a guide, the authors use Baker's classification of neck aging, which grades progressive aging from I to IV.[52] Class III patients with moderate cervical skin laxity and poor neck skin elasticity (usually in their late 50s–60s) and class IV patients with severe deep skin neck laxity and folds below the level of the cricoid (usually in their late 60s–70s) are most at risk for the mandibular ligaments limiting neck skin redraping.

VERTICAL NECK LIFT TECHNIQUE

The following is a description of the authors' vertical neck lifting procedure. This technique is an extended deep plane facelift, which elevates the skin and SMAS-platysma complex as a composite unit. The goal is to redrape cervicomental laxity vertically onto the face rather than laterally and postauricularly. The authors consider this an extended technique because it lengthens the deep plane flap from the angle of the mandible, as originally described by Hamra,[21] into the

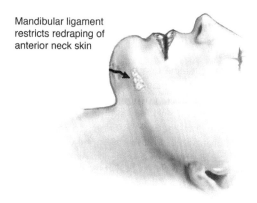

Mandibular ligament restricts redraping of anterior neck skin

Fig. 7. Tethering of the mandibular ligament along the anterior mandible limits mobilization and redraping of the anterior submental skin directly beneath it in patients with more redundant neck skin.

neck to release the cervical retaining ligaments that limit platysmal redraping. It also includes release of the zygomatic and mandibular retaining ligaments to allow for greater vertical neck elevation. This technique does not routinely use midline platysmal surgery because it counteracts the extent of vertical redraping. A majority of aging face patients are good candidates for this procedure in isolation, but indications for combining vertical neck lifting with submental surgery are elucidated later.

INDICATIONS AND ANCILLARY PROCEDURES

Preoperative evaluation for the vertical neck lift begins with a through physical examination. This examination includes observing how the face and neck redrapes when traction is placed on the skin along the vertical vectors consistent with this neck lifting technique. The senior author has had success with patients ages 40 to 70 years, even in the presence of significant anterior platysmal cording and submental skin excess.

This dynamic physical examination technique can be used to determine candidacy for an isolated vertical neck lift without midline platysmoplasty. It involves traction on the facial skin along the deep plane entry point line to evaluate the vertical and horizontal components of the neck (**Fig. 8**).

- The surgeon places 3 fingers at the deep plane entry point line, from the angle of the mandible to the lateral canthus, on both sides of the face and moves the skin vertically to assess whether the submental platysmal and skin laxity is corrected.

- If patients still have significant neck redundancy with this maneuver and platysmal cording exists, then a midline platysmaplasty should be planned in addition to the vertical neck lift.

Another guideline used when deciding whether to add a platysmaplasty to the vertical neck lift procedure is based on anatomic studies. These studies demonstrated that extending a traditional deep plane rhytidectomy inferiorly to release the cervical retaining ligaments achieves greater lateral motion of the midline platysma. The average redraping of the midline platysma is 2.4 cm with the extended technique.[47] Given these findings, the authors typically perform a midline platysmoplasty when the platysmal divergence approaches 3 cm.

There are several options that have been created to address the neck and submentum

from the midline. These include the sideways-type overlap of the upper medial platysma by Boo and Woodsmith[53] and later by Fuente Del Campo.[54] A vest-over-pants technique has been described by Guyuron and colleagues,[55] but the authors prefer a method similar to the original corsette platysmaplasty described by Feldman.[56]

There are anatomic variants that should be noted on physical examination that predispose to failures and require combining direct submental techniques with the vertical neck lift. These include presence of excessive supraplatysmal and subplatysmal fat, digastric muscle hypertrophy, low anterior hyoid, submandibular gland ptosis, and retrognathia. Excessive supraplatysmal fat may require liposuction or excision. Midline subplatysmal dissection allows for direct excision and treatment of excess subplatysma fat, and anterior digastrics may be addressed by partial/full excision or plication.

Patients possessing a low hyoid or short neck may prove be the most difficult to treat. Excision of the anterior portion of the hyoid has also been advocated in the treatment of a low-lying hyoid in certain instances.[55] Prominence of the submandibular glands should also be assessed. Although some investigators advocate partial or complete excision to decrease fullness in this region, this has not been an issue during rhytidectomy performed by the senior author. This may in part be due to the vertical suspension of the platysma surrounding the glands, which opposes the ptosis or descent, which has been shown to occur with aging.[57] There are also conflicting data about the efficacy of submandibular gland reduction techniques, with some studies showing that the complications may be worse than the improvement[58] and that improvements are uncertain.[3,59] Lastly, if retrognathia is present, this may limit the degree of improvement visualized after the neck lift. By increasing the length of the jaw with chin augmentation, the perceived depth of the cervicomental angle is enhanced on profile.[60–62]

SURGICAL TECHNIQUE
Preoperative Marking

The patient is positioned upright preoperatively and important landmarks are drawn with a marking pen (**Fig. 9**). The path of the temporal branch of the facial nerve is marked beginning at the root of the ear lobule, traversing at a point halfway between the lateral canthus and tragus, and ending approximately 1.5 cm from the lateral brow. Next the deep plane entry point is marked as a line

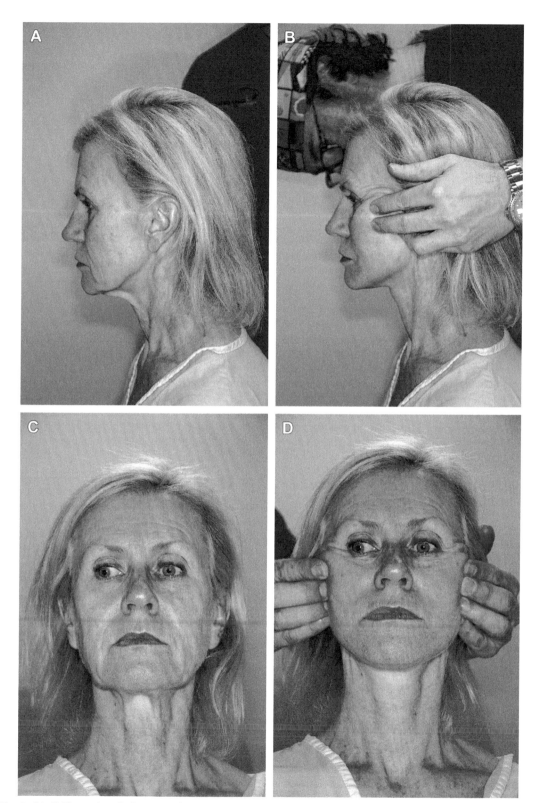

Fig. 8. (*A, B*) The patient is shown undergoing the authors' preoperative maneuver demonstrating how the anticipated vertical vector elevation along a deep plane entry point in the face treats platysmal cording and submental laxity. For this part of the examination, the surgeon places 3 fingers at the deep plane entry point (*line coursing from the angle of the mandible to the lateral canthus*) on both sides of the face and moves the skin vertically to assess whether the submental and platysmal skin laxity is corrected with this tension. (*C, D*) Views of the submental region with preoperative maneuver. If the submental area is corrected, no anterior platysmal surgery is necessary. If patients still have platysmal redundancy, a midline corset platysmaplasty should concomitantly be performed.

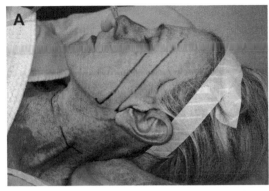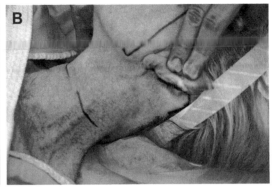

Fig. 9. (A) Preauricular and (B) postauricular rhytidectomy incision markings. Note the temporal hair tuft sparing incision with extension superiorly to allow for vertical skin elevation.

extending from the angle of the mandible to the lateral canthus. The perimandibular skin is mobilized to identify the where the mandibular ligament tethers the perijowl and submental neck skin and is marked. A submental incision is marked at the submental crease. Incision lines are then drawn beginning in the anterior temporal hairline typically at the height of the lateral brow. This incision follows around the temporal tuft and into the hairless recess between the sideburn and helical root, turning downward into the preauricular crease, paralleling the curve of the helical margin and approximately at the width of the of the crus of the helix. This incision is similar to that described by other investigators[63] with several minor modifications. In a majority of patients, the incision proceeds in a retrotragal manner, just along the posterior margin of the tragus. For male patients, the authors discuss the potential for posterior beard hairline transposition with this approach and allow them to decide. The incision then continues in a counterclockwise manner down the lobule-facial crease and around the lobule onto the posterior conchal cartilage skin to the level of the triangular fossa. In patients with greater neck skin laxity, the incision transitions down and follows the anterior edge of the occipital hairline several centimeters, depending on the anticipated amount of cervical skin resection.

Anesthesia

The senior author performs rhytidectomy under local anesthesia, conscious sedation, or general anesthesia solely based on patient preference. Approximately 20% of these patients elect to receive only local anesthesia, typically for financial reasons or fear of general anesthesia, whereas the remaining patients choose to receive local anesthesia with intravenous sedation with proprofol. A mixture of 50 mL of 1% lidocaine with 1:100,000 units of epinephrine, 50 mL of 0.25% bupivacaine with 1:200,000 units of epinephrine, 50 mL of 0.9% sodium chloride is used. If performed under local anesthesia, 15 mL of 8.4% sodium bicarbonate is added as well. This mixture provides a rapid-onset, long-duration, adequate hemostasis and greater comfort given the inclusion of buffer. Tissue resistance is noted during injection because it provides a preview of how easily the tissue planes will dissect and the extent of ligamentous attachments throughout the cervicofacial region.

Incision and Skin Flap Elevation

Skin incision is initiated at the anterior temporal hairline at the level of the lateral brow with a no. 10 scalpel cutting perpendicular to the skin. This can be extended superiorly during the operation if needed to redrape and remove the vertically elevated skin. In the past, the authors implemented a beveled, trichophytic incision but noted depression of the incision in a significant percentage of cases. The authors believe this occurs because the skin of the anterior temporal region is thin and the skived edge of the beveled incision tends to become devitalized and heal in a contracted fashion. This is different from the thicker anterior forehead/scalp skin in the area of the frontal hairline where trichophytic incisions were first described. The authors have noted temporal scars that are barely perceptible with this modification (**Fig. 10**).

- The incision is then carried down the preauricular path (described previously). The incision should not be placed at the anterior edge of the helical crus cartilage because it can make the root of the helix appear unnaturally wide. It should be placed at the natural highlight, which reflects the apparent width of the helical crus.

- The incision should then traverse along the posterior edge of the tragus but not on its inner

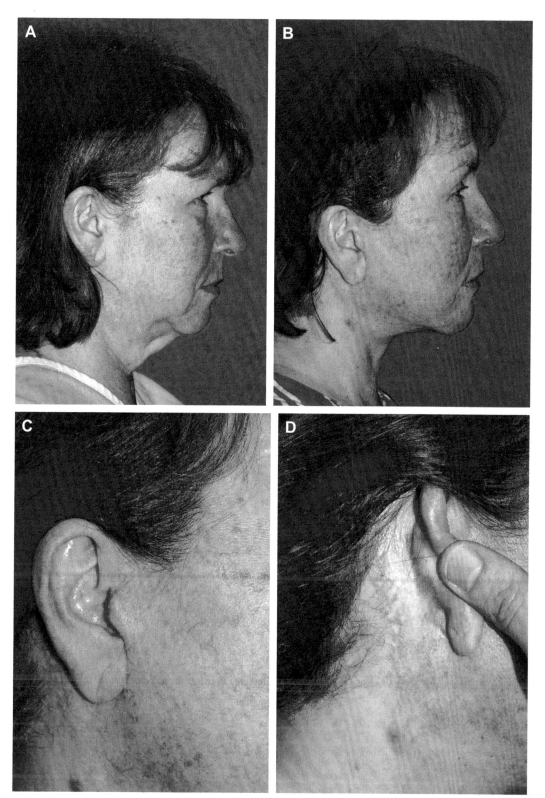

Fig. 10. (*A*) Preoperative lateral view of 57-year-old woman seeking neck rejuvenation; (*B*) 8-month postoperative lateral view after vertical neck lift. (*C*) Preauricular and extended anterior temporal incision and (*D*) postauricular incision not perceptible at 8 months.

surface because this can create an unnatural folding of the cheek skin that blunts the tragus and can be a telltale sign of a facelift incision A small step in the incision is placed at the inferior tragus to preserve the inferior tragal border (**Fig. 11**).

Around the earlobe, the incision should continue 2 mm inferior to the lobule cheek junction to preserve the natural sulcus between the lobe and the cheek.

- Posteriorly, the incision should continue a few millimeters onto the posterior conchal cartilage rather than directly in the postauricular crease. This helps minimize later inferior descent of the posterior auricular scar into a more visible location with age.

- In patients with less neck laxity, the incision ends here. If a surgeon is uncertain of the amount of neck skin that needs excision, the incision can always be extended to remove redundancy.

- In cases of more significant neck skin excess, the incision is transitioned at the level of the triangular fossa down the anterior aspect of the occipital hairline posteroinferiorly. Here the authors use a beveled trichophytic incision because the scalp skin is thicker here and the attendant problems (discussed previously) have not been noted. In the past, the authors used a high transverse incision that was hidden into the occipital hair. To prevent hairline margin step-offs, this incision requires that the neck skin flap be shifted anteriorly and vertically,

which limits the amount of redundant neck skin that can be removed (**Fig. 12**).

- The length of the incision in the occipital region depends on the amount of cervical skin to be excised in the posterior flap. The authors prefer to be conservative with the initial length of this incision to limit scarring, because it can always be extended to remove a dog-ear deformity.

- The initial portion of the subcutaneous flap is then elevated using a Brown-Adson forceps and a no. 10 scalpel beginning with the superior preauricular point. The plane should be elevated just deep to the reticular dermis leaving a very thin layer of fat attached to the flap. The temporal region skin is elevated with a broad, parallel stroke of the blade for 2 cm.

- After elevating the 2-cm skin pocket, the flap is able to accommodate an Anderson multiple-prong retractor. This is used to place superior and lateral tension on the flap.

- Direct countertension is placed by an assistant manually retracting the skin in the opposite direction and the flap is backlit with an operating room light to visualize the subdermal plexus.

- Flap elevation continues with facelift scissors, tips pointed upward, making small, forward-snipping motions to create an even-thickness flap. The intensity of the transilluminated light gives the surgeon the ability to gauge the thickness of the flap and create a uniform thickness.

- Elevation in the cheek ends at the marked line of the deep plane entry point (**Fig. 13**).

- The postauricular skin is then grasped at its postauricular peak with a Brown-Adson forceps and sharp dissection with a no. 10 blade is carried inferiorly. The skin in this region has a paucity of subcutaneous fat and is tightly adherent to the fascia overlying the SCM and mastoid so blade dissection is more expedient.

- Sharp dissection continues inferiorly to the level of the angle of the mandible and connects to the anteriorly created cheek subcutaneous flap.

- At this point, inferior and medial dissection in the neck in a subcutaneous/supraplatysmal plane is accomplished with a lighted retractor to provide tension while vertical-blunt spreading with a facelift scissors.

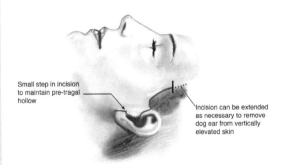

Small step in incision to maintain pre-tragal hollow

Incision can be extended as necessary to remove dog ear from vertically elevated skin

Fig. 11. Preauricular retrotragal incision in the vertical neck lift. The temporal hair tuft incision is extended anteriorly and superiorly to the level of the lateral brow to enable excision in the temporal region without hairline displacement. Also, note small step in the incision is placed at the inferior tragus to preserve the inferior tragal border.

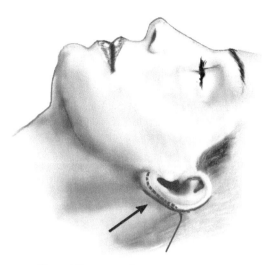
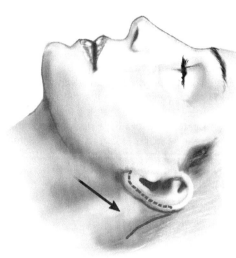

Flap shift to match
hairline limits
anterior neck
redraping

Flap shift perpendicular
to incision redrapes
neck redundancy
most effectively

Fig. 12. Postauricular incision. (*A*) Occipital hairline incision allows for greater neck skin redundancy excision because the neck skin flap can be redraped, without concern for hairline step-offs, perpendicular to the incision. (*B*) High transverse incision hidden into the occipital hair requires that the neck skin flap be shifted anteriorly and vertically to match the hairline and prevent hairline step-offs. This neck skin flap shift limits the amount of redundant neck skin that can be removed.

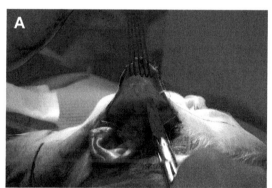
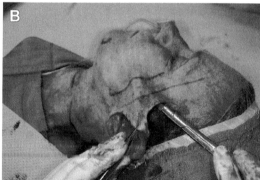
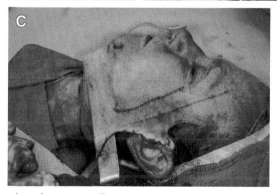

Fig. 13. (*A*) Transilluminating the subcutaneous flap and advancing with small snips at the level of the light-dark interface creates a flap of uniform thickness at the subdermal plexus. (*B*) In the cheek, the subcutaneous flap is elevated to the deep plane entry point. (*C*) In the neck, the subcutaneous flap is elevated to midline and inferiorly to just below the cricoid cartilage in the fascial plane just superficial to the platysma muscle.

Dissecting inferiorly over the SCM in this manner preserves the great auricular nerve, which courses from the posterior border of the SCM anterosuperiorly to the region of the lobule. Dissecting on top of the supraplatysma fascia with the medial neck skin elevation preserves a blanket of fat on the skin flap that prevents irregularities and adhesions between the deep dermis of the skin and the platysma postoperatively. This dissection is continued to the midline using a longer lighted retractor and long facelift scissors and extending inferiorly just below the level of the cricoid. This pocket will be connected to the opposite side when it is elevated.

Deep Plane and Prezygomatic Space Dissection

- An Anderson 5-prong retractor is placed at the anterior extent of the cheek skin subcutaneous elevation, and the flap is held under significant vertical tension away from the body.

- A no. 10 scalpel is used to make an incision into the deep plane (**Fig. 14**). The tension facilitates entry into the sub-SMAS–subplatysma complex.

- The incision starts at angle of the mandible and ultimately extends to the lateral canthus.

- For approximately 3 cm superior to the angle of the mandible, the platysma fibers can be visualized and are penetrated entering the sub-SMAS plane that appears as a glistening white fascial layer.

- A lighted retractor is again used to create vertical tension away from the body and vertical blunt dissection with facelift scissors helps elevate the composite skin and platysma flap off of the parotideomasseteric fascia (**Fig. 15**). The platysma undersurface is easily visible and dissection of this plane can proceed with finger dissection.

- The anterior extent of this dissection is to the level of the facial artery, which can be palpated and visualized in this plane.

- Elevation of this flap continues superiorly until resistance is reached at the zygomatic osteocutaneous ligaments.

Surgical note
To allow for vertical elevation of the SMAS, platysma, and skin with the authors' vertical neck lift technique, the zygomatic-cutaneous ligaments must be freed or bunching occurs in the lateral periorbital region. This also allows for more significant improvement in the midface by vertically repositioning the malar fat pad. Without cheek retaining ligament release, the melolabial fold and cheek remain in a heavy, gravitated position. Ultimately, failure to mobilize the malar ligament prevents adequate redistribution of the entire SMAS-platysma complex.

- *Isolation of the ligaments begins with blunt dissection at the superior extent of the deep plane entry point, creating a plane superficial to the orbicularis oculi muscle. This plane is contiguous with the prezygomatic space that is superficial to the zygomaticus musculature of the face.[45] The prezygomatic space can be easily dissected with blunt finger dissection medially to free it to the nasal facial crease. This technique was originally described as finger-assisted malar elevation by Aston (**Fig. 16**).[64,65]*

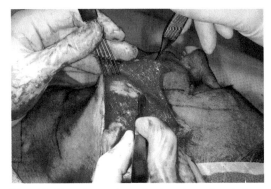

Fig. 14. The deep plane is sharply entered from the angle of the mandible to the lateral canthus with a no. 10 blade while applying tension on the face at the deep plane entry point with a 5-prong retractor.

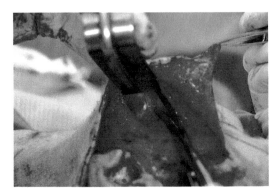

Fig. 15. The deep plane is developed with blunt vertical scissor dissection minimizing any risk to facial nerves while flap elevation proceeds.

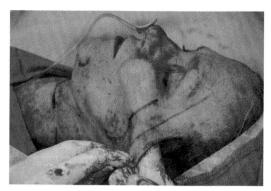

Fig. 16. The prezygomatic space is easily dissected superior to the zygomatic cutaneous ligaments with blunt finger dissection to the nasofacial groove.

Release of the Zygomatic Cutaneous Ligaments

The zygomatic osteocutaneous ligaments are now intervening between the cheek dissected superiorly in the prezygomatic space and inferiorly in the sub-SMAS plane. These ligaments tether the SMAS-platysma complex to the malar bone and prevent vertical elevation of the flap.

- Sharp dissection of the ligaments is initiated with a no. 10 scalpel. Dissecting from superior to inferior protects any facial nerve branches that enter the zygomaticus musculature from inferior and deep (**Fig. 17**).

- Once the densest portion of the ligaments has been severed sharply, blunt dissection continues on the surface of the zygomaticus major and minor until reaching the nasolabial fold medially overlying the zygoma. This has been defined as the premaxillary space, and a dense maxillary ligament that tethers the midface

is bluntly dissected to further release the midface.[45]

Release of the Cervical Retaining Ligaments

With the deep plane now free, the only remaining point that tethers the SMAS-platysma complex from moving vertically is the cervical retaining ligaments.

- Through the inferior aspect of the deep plane flap, the platysma is elevated inferiorly below the margin of the mandible for approximately 5 cm with tension of the flap with a lighted retractor away from the body and continued vertical scissor spreading blunt dissection (**Fig. 18**).

- The tips of the scissors are spread into the fascia underlying the platysma, leaving the marginal mandibular and cervical branches of the facial nerve down on the superficial cervical fascia that is contiguous with the parotid-masseteric fascia.

- The dissection proceeds inferiorly and posteriorly in a backhanded direction to free the platysma except at its posterior attachment to the SCM investing fascia or the cervical retaining ligaments.

- With the extended inferior platysma dissection completed, a marking pen is used to draw the lateral platysmal border at its connection to the SCM for 5 cm below the angle of the mandible extending the deep plane inferiorly.

- A no. 15 scalpel is used to make a broad and gentle incision until a lip of tissue is obtained, the edge grasped, and sharp dissection within

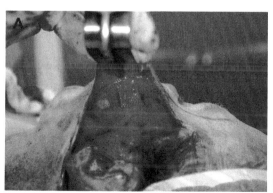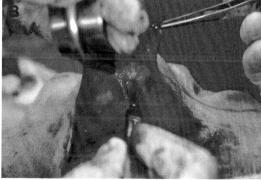

Fig. 17. (*A*) The dense zygomatic cutaneous ligament is isolated after blunt dissection of the deep plane inferiorly and superiorly. (*B*) Sharp dissection through the densest part of the ligament with a no. 10 blade superiorly to inferiorly protects any facial nerve branches that enter the zygomaticus musculature from inferior and deep.

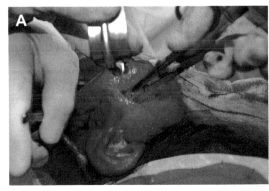
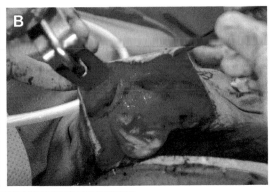
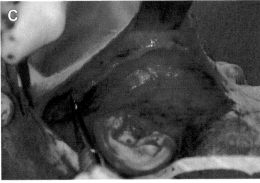

Fig. 18. (*A*) The deep plane is extended below the angle of the mandible into the neck by bluntly dissecting in the subplatymsa plane form the inferior aspect of the deep plane pocket developed in the cheek. (*B*) The platysma is sharply released from its LATERAL attachments to the SCM EXTENDING 5 cm below the angle of the mandible, as shown by the extent of the marking. (*C*) The extended deep plane flap after release is shown.

the SCM fascia is continued for approximately 1 cm.

- A lighted retractor is then placed under the lip, retracting away from the body, and a facelift scissor is used to bluntly dissect through the ligaments and the area of the subplatysma flap previously elevated is freed.

Deep Plane Flap Suspension

- A cuff or lip of platysma/SMAS is separated at the deep plane entry point for placement of suspension sutures.

- Facelift scissors are used with small snips along the entire deep plane entry point.

- Irrigation is performed with a bacitracin solution and hemostasis obtained with bipolar electrocautery to minimize thermal injury to flaps and any nerves.

At dissection's end, the result from inferior to superior should be a platysma-SMAS complex free on the superior, inferior, and deep borders that can be mobilized without restriction vertically.

- The SMAS and platysma are conjoined to the skin as a composite flap from the mandibular border until the orbital rim, and skin is freed as cutaneous flaps in the temporal region as well as in the neck below the angle of the mandible and postauricular region.

- The deep plane flap is typically sutured at 3 nearly equidistant points along the cuff formed from angle to lateral canthus.

- The flap is suspended at an angle that tightens the tissues into the cervicomental angle, which is parallel to an imaginary line that bisects the angle.

Surgical note

Individual anatomy dictates this angle, differing in those with a low- versus a high-positioned hyoid or in patients with a short versus long mandible. On average, this angle approaches 60° in many patients. When examining the vectors of redraping in more than 300 patients, this angle varies from the upper 40°s to 70°s. Still, the angle is always more vertical than an exact superolateral vector of 45°.[23]

- *The first suture (3-0 nylon, PS-2 needle) is placed in a horizontal mattress fashion from the cuff created at the deep plane entry point to the parotid masseteric fascia in the pretragal (or preauricular) region but is left untied for the moment (Fig. 19).*

- *The 2 remaining sutures are thrown similarly, yet their vectors tend to become slightly less vertical as they progress superiorly. The most superior suture is suspended to the deep temporal fascia.*

Mandibular Ligament Release

Before tying the deep plane suspension sutures, redraping of the anterior submental skin is noted as the deep plane flap is elevated vertically. In patients with more significant neck skin redundancy, the mandibular ligaments may tether the skin at the mandibular border preventing anterior submental skin tightening. The tethering effect of the mandibular ligaments is variable and depends on their elasticity and position. In some patients, the mandibular ligaments have greater flexibility or elasticity and their tethering effect is less significant. They have the greatest distensibility of all the facial retaining ligaments in biomechanical studies.[50] Additionally, the further posterior the ligament is displaced from the symphyisis the greater tethering effect it has in the neck.

Successful implementation involves identification of mandibular ligament location with dynamic examination used to locate the greatest point of tethering. The authors have noted this point to be on average 5 cm lateral to the symphysis in examination of 75 patients.[52] Identification of the correct zone can be performed by distracting the skin along the anterior aspect of the mandible away from the face.

- The area of tethering should be drawn with a marking pen.

- The approach is through a submental incision of approximately 2 cm.

- A Brown-Adson forceps is used for skin retraction and a subcutaneous dissection ensues using a sharp iris scissors.

- Full release of the ligaments requires dissection to the posterior edge of the tethering point and inferiorly to the lower edge of the mandible as it transitions to neck (Fig. 20).

Surgical note
The marginal branch of the facial nerve has been shown to exist posterior to the ligament in studies by Langevin and colleagues,[51] so it is not at risk during this dissection.

Lateral Platymsa Suspension in the Neck

Once the decision has been made to release the mandibular ligament and the deep plane flap has been suspended and tied, the platysma flap below the mandibular angle is addressed. With vertical repositioning of the deep plane flap, the redundant platysma overlies the auricle, and the platymsa must be split at the level of the ear lobule so that redraping of the platysma can occur postauricularly. A horizontal myotomy parallel to the inferior margin of the mandible at the horizontal platysmal border allows for this to occur (Fig. 21).

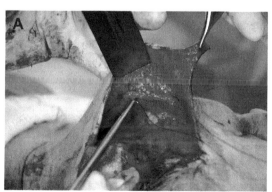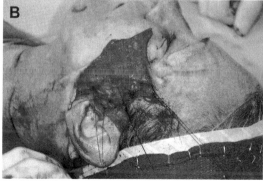

Fig. 19. (A) To suspend the deep plane flap, a cuff is developed with scissor dissection at the deep plane entry point. Here, horizontal mattress 3-0 nylon sutures are placed. (B) The sutures placed in the flap are sutured to deep anchoring points in the preauricular and temporal region after choosing the proper vertical vector for redraping.

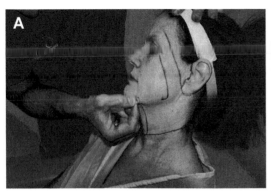
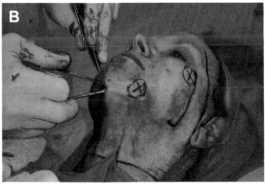
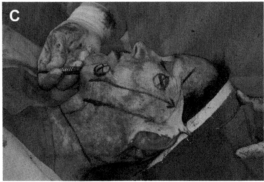

Fig. 20. (*A*) The tethering of the mandibular ligament on the anterior neck can be assessed preoperatively by distracting the skin along the anterior one-third of the jawline. (*B*) The mandibular ligament can be released in a subcutaneous plane from a submental incision. Release extends from the anterior aspect of the mandible inferiorly to below the inferior mandibular border. (*C*) Maximal anterior submental skin redraping is shown after release and vertical redraping of the facelift flap along a vector that parallels a line that bisects the cervicomental angle. Release of the mandibular ligament is demonstrated with an instrument placed in the submental incision.

- An approximately 3-cm myotomy is made at the level of the angle of the mandible.

- After myotomy, the inferior platysmal tab is anchored with a 3-0 nylon suture vertically to the mastoid tip.

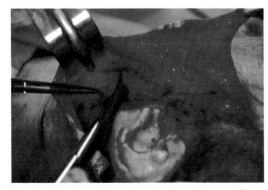

Fig. 21. A horizontal myotomy in the platysmal flap is made at the level of the angle of the mandible to redrape the platysma vertically to the mastoid tip. The platysma is sutured to the mastoid.

Surgical note
This vector of pull is transmitted along submandibular region directly away from the cervicomental angle. This maneuver creates definition at the posterior mandibular border and angle. Plication of the platysma in this region without flap elevation and redraping often creates an unnatural fullness in the area just below the angle of the mandible due to bunching.

- *Typically 2 more sutures are placed inferior to the platysmal tab approximately 2 cm apart to redrape the released platysma flap to the SCM.*

- *A Jackson-Pratt drain is then placed from the hairline into the neck until the next morning to decrease bruising and recovery time.*

- *Once the SMAS-platysma complex is suspended, the skin is then redraped.*

Surgical note
In the cheek and face, the same plane must be used because a composite flap was elevated along

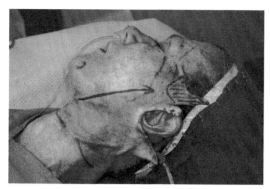

Fig. 22. A majority of the neck skin is removed in the anterior temporal region due to the vertical redraping of the flap.

the majority of the facial rhytidectomy. A majority of the skin is removed vertically in the temporal region (Fig. 22). Because the skin has been delaminated from the platysma in the neck, redraping of the neck skin can be mobilized independently for the best contour.

- Excess skin is then removed segmentally at all points from anterior to posterior after suturing. Adequate elevation of the temporal skin in the subcutaneous plane avoids bunching.

- In those patients with more significantly laxity, the temporal incision must be carried superior to the lateral brow to correct a dog-ear.

- Deep everting 4-0 Vicryl sutures are placed along the entire temporal incision to prevent depression and spreading of the scar over time. The authors encountered more obvious anterior temporal scars when the vertical neck lifting technique using only a superficial skin closure was first adopted.

- Skin closure is with everting 5-0 nylon vertical mattress sutures.

- The remainder of the incision is closed with 5-0 nylon sutures anteriorly, 5-0 nylon sutures behind the ear, and 4-0 nylon in the occipital hairline (Fig. 23).

- The submental incision is then closed if present and a head wrap is placed until the next morning only.

- A majority of anterior sutures are removed at 4 days.

Adjunctive Submental Procedures and Platysmoplasty

If the need for an additional midline submental procedure is confirmed preoperatively, the authors perform this first prior to lifting the neck skin and platysma portion. Increasing the number of procedures performed in the submentum increases the chances of irregularities, and each maneuver must be performed precisely and in a metered fashion.

The authors perform subcutaneous liposuction in the neck in fewer than 5% of patients and only when they have significant supraplatysmal fat excess, which can be grasped and clearly identified prior to injection. An approximate guideline for performing submental liposuction is when more than 3 cm of thickness can be grasped in the submental skin between the thumb and forefinger. In cases of liposuction needed for improved cervical contour, this precedes any platysmal work through a small incision in the submental crease to maintain adequate suction. In general, the authors prefer to leave the natural blanket of fat between the skin and platysma to avoid forming depressions from adhesions and retraction. Adequate release and redraping, as described with the vertical neck lifting technique, most often obviates submental liposuction. When performing submental liposuction, the authors use modern techniques

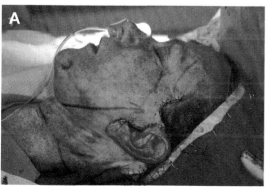
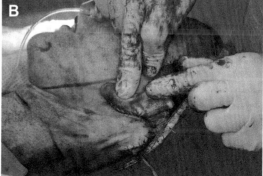

Fig. 23. (A) Preauricular skin closure. (B) Posterior auricular skin closure.

that mitigate the chance of commonly noted irregularities.[66–75] Removal of fat at and above the jawline and jowls is avoided because there is a greater chance of iatrogenic irregularity here. The authors no longer use large spatulated cannulae to avoid skeletonization, retraction, and fibrosis. Instead, the authors use small microliposuction cannulae to decrease the chance of lumps and bumps postoperatively.

- With the suction off the cannula, a preplatysmal plane is dissected in the neck.

- The cannula is then placed on suction and supraplatysmal fat is removed with the opening pointed toward the platysma, taking great care to leave approximately 1 cm of protective fat layer on the dermis to avoid irregularities in this region. This thickness can be determined by rolling the skin between the thumb and index finger. The authors do not advocate the use of ultrasonic cannulae because the risk of thermal injury is higher.

- If subplatysmal fat excess must be addressed, the authors perform it in conjunction with a midline playsmoplasty.

- When removing subplatysmal fat, it is important to create a platysma corset in the midline to prevent adhesions and retraction between the skin and mylohyoid.

The vector of pull the authors use obviates midline platysma plication in a high percentage of cases. As demonstrated in cadaveric studies, a more vertical pull typically avoids distraction and dehiscence of the midline platysma seen with a superolateral vector of pull.[26] Although there are a variety of platysmal grading scales and anatomic classifications available to assist in the selection procedure type,[52,55,76,77] the senior author uses midline platysmal procedures in cases of a tighter submental suspension necessary because of excessive platysmal redundancy or when there is excessive banding or dehiscence present.

The decision to perform a midline platysma corset is usually made preoperatively. As discussed previously, the 2 primary indicators for including a platysmoplasty are (1) the preoperative physical examination noting inadequate neck redraping when the facial tissues are lifted vertically along the deep plane entry point and (2) platysmal dehiscence approaching 3 cm. The authors have noted the need for midline platysma corset surgery in only 13% of patients. The authors prefer to make this determination preoperatively and perform this medial work prior to the lift because it is difficult to reapproximate the midline platysmal edges after they have been lifted vertically with the extended deep plane release and resuspension of the platysma. With this in mind, the decision to perform the midline corset can also be made intraoperatively when midline platysma laxity is noted after elevation and redraping of the lateral platysma flaps with the vertical neck lift.

The type of platysmaplasty performed is similar to the corset platysmaplasty described by Feldman,[56] with minor modifications. Feldman originally described extensive defatting in nearly all zones of the neck, making the incision in the submentum after the face had already been dissected and only excising the intraplatysmal fibers when the platysma is decussated below the chin.

- The authors only perform a smaller submental incision (typically 2 cm), elevating the neck skin in a supraplatysmal fascial plane using blunt vertical spreads with a facelift scissors to a level just below the cricoid cartilage.

- The intraplatysmal fibers are then clamped with a curved Kelly clamp and the tissues below the clamp are resected with a no. 15 scalpel and then cauterized in a method similar to that described by other investigators.[78]

- At this point, the subplatysmal fat and digastric muscles are examined and the need for reduction is determined.

- Subplastymal flaps are elevated laterally to the submandibular gland anterior border to assist in mobilization and to decrease the chance of palpable midline banding.

- Because postoperative dehiscence has been noted in prior experience, the authors prefer permanent sutures and place interrupted and buried 3-0 nylon. Burying the knots helps minimize the possibility of palpation of the sutures through the skin.

DISCUSSION

Although there are a plethora of techniques used for face and neck lifting, the authors have evolved to a vertical vector, extended deep plane approach described herein to address the pitfalls inherent to neck lifting surgery, the most common of which are either inadequate neck tightening or early postoperative neck ptosis (**Figs. 24** and **25**).

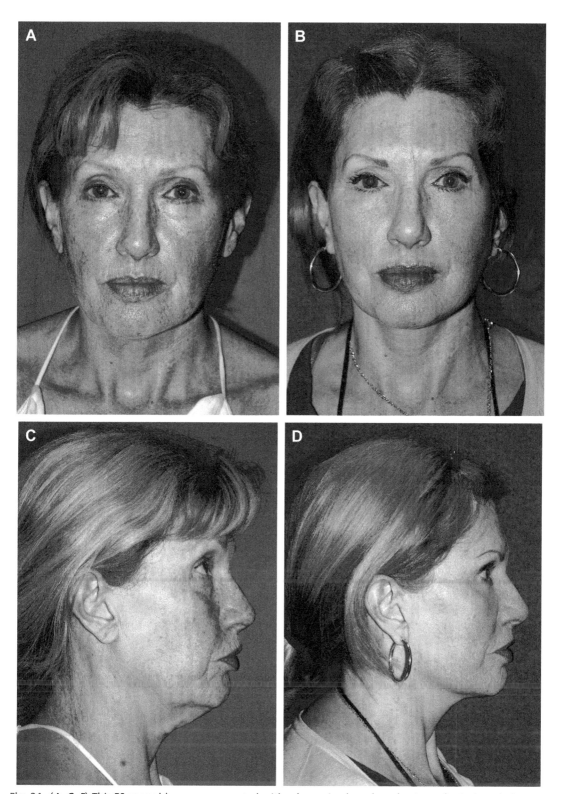

Fig. 24. (*A, C, E*) This 59-year-old woman presented with a heavy jowls and moderate neck ptosis and platysma laxity and was a candidate for a vertical neck lift without midline platysmal surgery. (*B, D, F*) Seventeen months after vertical neck lift using the authors' extended deep plane rhytidectomy approach, including mandibular ligament release. Note the complete correction of the platysmal banding and cervicomental laxity. She also had a lower blepharoplasty with fat transposition at the same time.

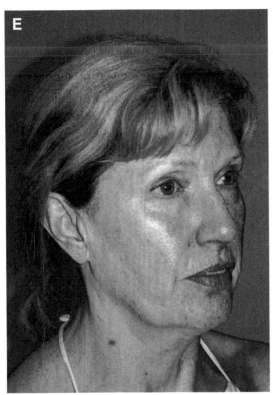
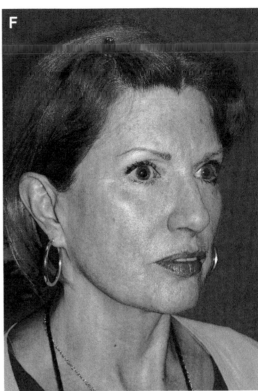

Fig. 24. (*continued*). (*E*) Preop with heavy jowls and moderate neck ptosis and platysma laxity. (*F*) Seventeen months after vertical neck lift using the authors' extended deep plane rhytidectomy approach, including mandibular ligament release. She also had a lower blepharoplasty with fat transposition at the same time.

The challenge is achieving the planned outcome while avoiding the stigmata typically associated with an operated neck. These include irregularities in the submental region, such as depression and adherence of the skin to the platysma after cervical subcutaneous liposuction; suprahyoid depressions from subplatysmal fat excision; and suprahyoid fullness and bulkiness from repositioning the medial edges of the platysma muscle midline during corset platysmoplasty (**Fig. 26**). Because of frustration with neck irregularities encountered in a significant percentage of cases (5%–10%) when using midline procedures, the authors developed a lateral approach that helped circumvent these problems.

The vertical vector of lifting for both the SMAS-platysma complex and skin has been critical to maximize the capacity of this lateral approach. Cadaveric studies demonstrate not only that a more vertical vector of SMAS and platysma elevation provides a greater lift along the jawline/jowls compared with a superolateral vector of repositioning but also that vertical tightening decreases midline platysmal dehiscence whereas superolateral vectors increase platysmal dehiscence.[26] The increasing platysmal dehiscence in superolateral vector face and neck lifting is why platysmal corseting is almost mandatory with these techniques. Forgoing the midline corset avoids the counteractive pull into the center of the neck that further limits the ability to lift the neck soft tissue into the cervicomental angle.

The addition of release of the retaining ligaments that anchor the SMAS-platysma complex has allowed for more significant vertical redraping. The most important of these are the zygomatic osteocutaneous ligaments that bind the SMAS to the malar bone and the cervical retaining ligaments that bind the platysma to the SCM fascia. Release of the mandibular ligaments may be required in some cases to allow for more significant redraping of the anterior submental skin, but their limiting effect can be evaluated on a case-by-case basis intraoperatively. Release of these structures permits achievement of a greater aesthetic with improved redraping of skin and soft tissues. This helps avoid postoperative failures with less chance of lateral sweep, submalar depression,[18] persistent jowling, and deepening

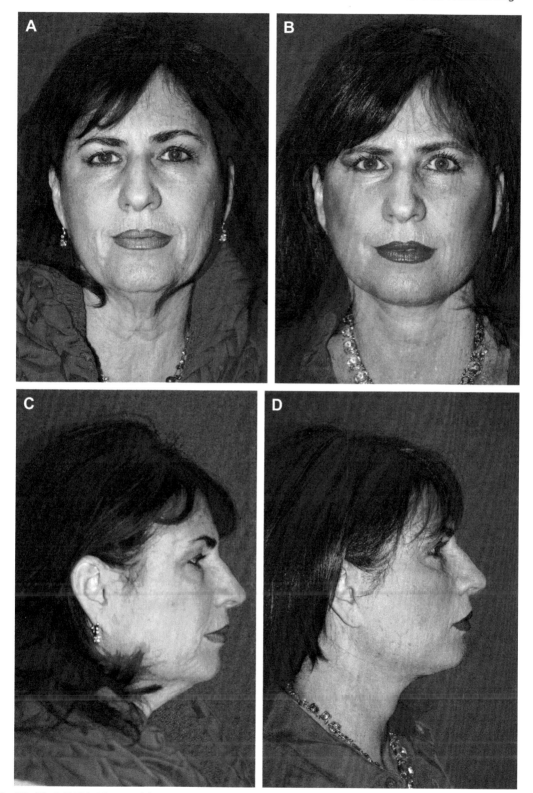

Fig. 25. (*A, C, E*) This 56-year-old woman presented with a heavy jowls, moderate neck ptosis, and platysma laxity, who was a candidate for a vertical neck lift without midline platysmal surgery. (*B, D, F*) Fifteen months after vertical neck lift using the authors' extended deep plane rhytidectomy approach, including mandibular ligament release. Note the complete correction of the platysmal banding and cervicomental laxity. She also had a lower blepharoplasty with fat transposition at the same time.

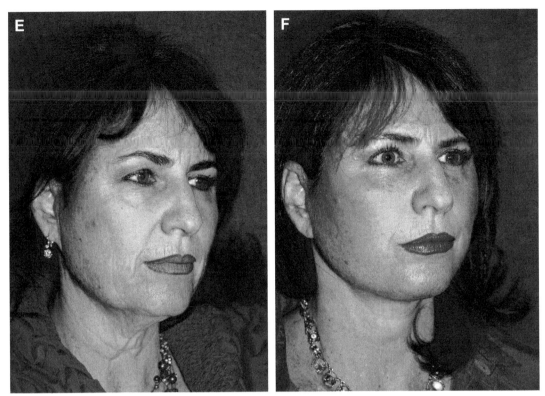

Fig. 25. (*continued*). (*E*) Heavy jowls, moderate neck ptosis, and platysma laxity. (*F*) Fifteen months after vertical neck lift using the authors' extended deep plane rhytidectomy approach, including mandibular ligament release. She also had a lower blepharoplasty with fat transposition at the same time.

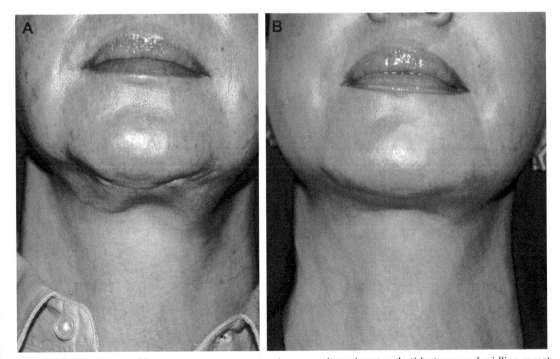

Fig. 26. (*A*) This 54-year-old woman was status post–prior superolateral vector rhytidectomy and midline corset platysmaplasty performed elsewhere 13 months earlier that resulted in submental fullness ad irregularities from pulling the bulk of the platysma midline and performing excessive submental liposuction. (*B*) Fourteen months after vertical reorientation facelift with release of the mandibular cutaneous ligaments. The greater deep plane release of the platysma allows for greater vertical reorientation of the platysma fullness and mandibular ligament release allows for greater tightening of the submental skin into the cervicomental angle.

of stasis of the nasolabial fold along with other stigmata typically associated with more superficial ligament-preserving techniques. A deep plane technique further enhances the postoperative results by preventing hollowing typically noted at and above the jawline in the preparotid region (**Fig. 27**). This deformity is associated with extensive subcutaneous dissection, which traumatizes fat cells and causes necrosis.

Many surgeons may be hesitant to advance to extending the deep plane from the angle of the mandible into the neck when dissecting the platysma, but the authors believe that limiting this dissection may restrict the transmitted degree of deep tissue mobilization[47] and a higher recurrence of platysmal bands.[13,14,79] The extended deep plane technique has been shown to provide a 554% greater superolateral motion of the platysma compared with SMAS-plastyma purse-string suture techniques.[20]

Prior mantra held that the marginal branch of the facial nerve would be at greater risk with subplatysmal techniques in the region inferior to the angle of the mandible and into the neck.[37,80–84] Experience has taught that this is not the case. Many investigators cite the risks of neck rejuvenation and discourage platysmal undermining in many cases.[81,85–91] The authors believe, however, that extensive dissection in a subplatysmal plane in the neck is consistent and safe when performed with meticulous and careful blunt dissection in the correct plane. The authors' blunt dissection approach undermines the platysma from the deep plane flap already elevated, inferiorly into the neck, allowing for safe platysma elevation.

Failure to release the platysma from the cervical retaining ligaments in this manner may result in an unwanted recurrence of neck ptosis and need for neck revision.[12,48,92,93]

The question remains: Is there a benefit to performing an extended deep plane vertical neck lift with such extensive dissection? And, if so, does this increase the risk of facial nerve damage among other complications? The vertical neck lift the authors describe has created a durable

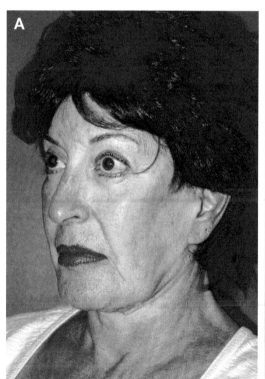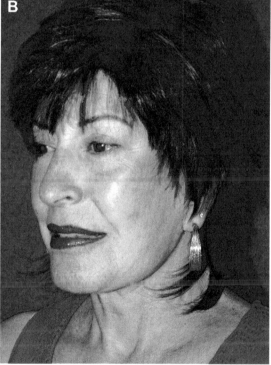

Fig. 27. (A) This 69-year-old woman was status post–prior rhytidectomy with subcutaneous skin flap and SMAS plication performed elsewhere 3 years earlier that resulted in subcutaneous atrophy in the region of the skin flap elevation; (B) 12 months after deep plane vertical face and neck lift. Effacement of this step-off where the prior skin flap ended is accomplished by releasing the entire cheek in the deep plane to the nasolabial fold and nasofacial crease and redraping vertically. She underwent a lateral retinacular suspension to correct lower eyelid retraction due to prior blepharoplasty.

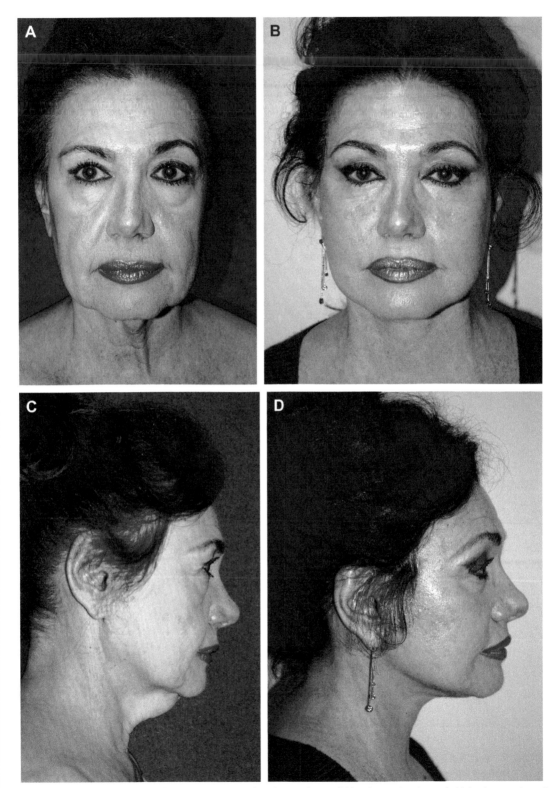

Fig. 28. (*A*, *C*, *E*) This 69-year-old woman presented with a turkey gobbler, heavy jowls, and thick platysmal cording and was not a candidate for a vertical neck lift without midline platysmal surgery. (*B*, *D*, *F*) Twelve months after vertical neck lift using the authors' extended deep plane rhytidectomy approach, including mandibular ligament release and midline platysmaplasty. Note the complete correction of the platysmal banding and cervicomental laxity.

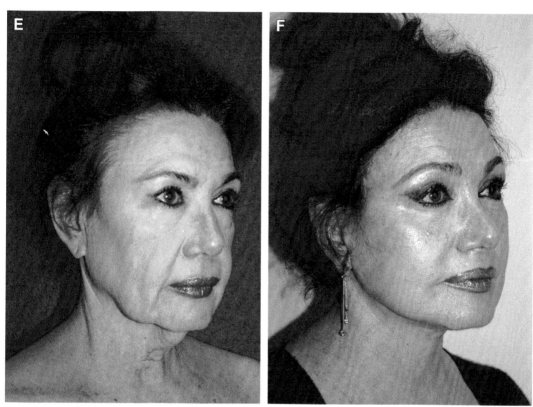

Fig. 28. (continued). (E) "Turkey gobbler," heavy jowls, and thick platysmal cording. (F) Twelve months after vertical neck lift using the authors' extended deep plane rhytidectomy approach, including mandibular ligament release and midline platysmaplasty. Complete correction of the platysmal banding and cervicomental laxity.

neck repair with a low tuck-up rate or need for additional submental improvement. Approximately one-third of revisions performed in the senior author's practice are on patients who had prior lateral SMASootomy or SMAS-platysma imbrication lifts elsewhere to address early recurrences of jowling and recurrent neck ptosis. Similar experiences have been reported elsewhere; Prado and colleagues[94] stated that more than 50% of patients undergoing MACS lift or lateral SMASectomy required a secondary tuck-up within 2 years. The superiority of deep plane techniques compared with more limited techniques, such as plication and imbrication, has been demonstrated intraoperatively with objective neck and jowl skin excision measurements.[47,95] Kamer demonstrated a 97% patient satisfaction rate in a cohort of 335 patients undergoing the deep plane technique, decreasing the tuck-up rate at 1 year to 3.3% compared with an 11.4% tuck-up rate with an extended SMAS flap cohort of 279 patients.[96] The authors' tuck-up rate in a prior series with the vertical neck

lifting technique was 3.1% for a cohort of 323 patients at 1 year.[49]

The authors' incidence of facial nerve injury with an extended deep plane approach is 1.2% in a prior study reviewing 323 patients who underwent this technique with the senior author.[49] This temporary facial nerve injury rate is the same as less-invasive SMAS plicating and suturing techniques that can cause temporary traction injury.[97]

With this approach, the need for corset platysmoplasty is not completely avoided. In the authors' experience of a review of 323 cases, 13% of patients had additional plastymal redundancy that required midline platysmal tightening in addition to the lateral approach (**Figs. 28 and 29**). These patients were usually in their late 60s and 70s, but the majority of patients presenting for rhytidectomy in their 50s and 60s did not require the additional submental approach.

Overall, the vertical neck lifting technique outlined in this article has been shown to provide durable neck rejuvenation while avoiding

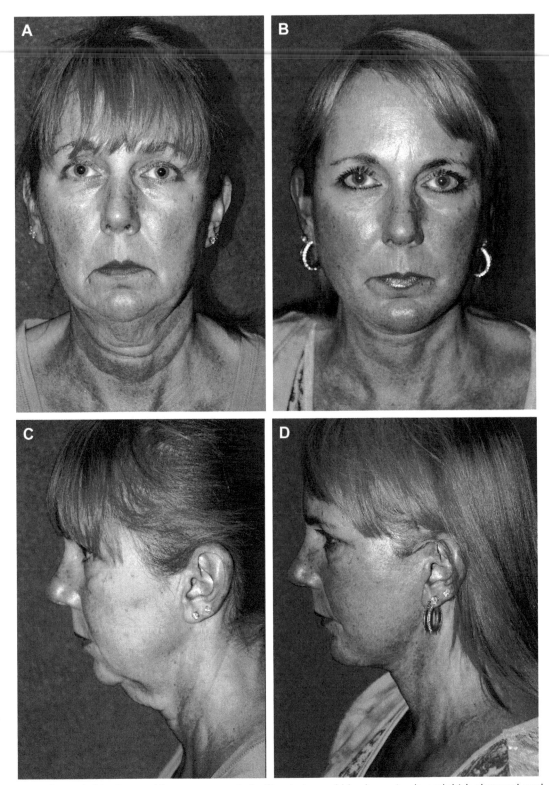

Fig. 29. (*A, C, E*) This 55-year-old woman presented with a turkey gobbler, heavy jowls, and thick platysmal cording and was not a candidate for a vertical neck lift without midline platysmal surgery. (*B, D, F*) Twelve months after vertical neck lift using the authors' extended deep plane rhytidectomy approach and midline platysmaplasty. Due to her retrognathia, she also required a chin implant executed through her submental incision. Placement of the chin implant releases the mandibular osteocutaneous ligaments in the subperiosteal plane. Note the complete correction of the platysmal banding and cervicomental laxity.

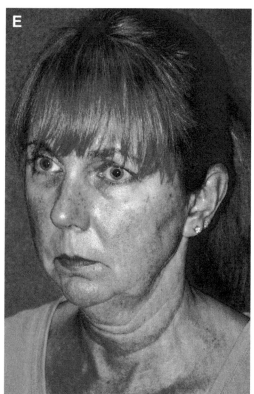
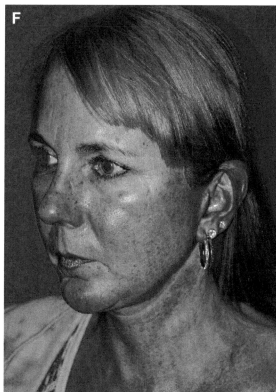

Fig. 29. (*continued*). (*E*) "Turkey gobbler," heavy jowls, and thick platysmal cordin. (*F*) Twelve months after vertical neck lift using the authors' extended deep plane rhytidectomy approach and midline platysmaplasty. Due to her retrognathia, she also required a chin implant executed through her submental incision.

submental surgery in a majority of cases. In the authors' experience, it seems to address the pitfalls typically associated with face and neck lifting while mitigating the risk for irregularities associated with ancillary submental procedures.

REFERENCES

1. Ellenbogen R, Karlin JV. Visual criteria for success in restoring the youthful neck. Plast Reconstr Surg 1980;66(6):826–37.
2. Okoog T. Plastic surgery: new methods and refinements. Philadelphia: Saunders; 1974. p. 310–30.
3. Mitz V, Peyronie M. The superficial musculoaponeurotic system (SMAS) in the parotid and cheek area. Plast Reconstr Surg 1976;58(1):80–8.
4. Connell BF. Pushing the clock back 15 to 20 years with facial rejuvenation. Clin Plast Surg 2008;35(4):553–66, vi.
5. Owsley JQ. Aesthetic facial surgery. St Louis (MO): Quality Medical; 1994.
6. Owsley JQ. Face lift. Plast Reconstr Surg 1997;100(2):514–9.
7. Barton FE. Facial rejuvenation. St Louis (MO): Quality Medical; 2008.
8. Baker TJ, Gordon HL, Stuzin JM. Surgical rejuvenation of the face. 2nd edition. St Louis (MO): Mosby; 1996.
0. Bakor TJ, Stuzin JM. Personal technique of face lifting. Plast Reconstr Surg 1997;100(2):502–8.
10. Stuzin JM. Restoring facial shape in face lifting: the role of skeletal support in facial analysis and midface soft-tissue repositioning. Plast Reconstr Surg 2007;119(1):362–76 [discussion: 377–8].
11. Stuzin JM, Baker TJ, Gordon HL, et al. Extended SMAS dissection as an approach to midface rejuvenation. Clin Plast Surg 1995;22(2):295–311.
12. Owsley JQ Jr. SMAS-platysma facelift. A bidirectional cervicofacial rhytidectomy. Clin Plast Surg 1983;10(3):429–40.
13. Baker DC. Lateral SMASectomy, plication and short scar facelifts: indications and techniques. Clin Plast Surg 2008;35(4):533–50, vi.
14. Tonnard P, Verpaele A. The MACS-lift short scar rhytidectomy. Aesthet Surg J 2007;27(2):188–98.
15. Hamra ST. Surgery of the aging chin. Plast Reconstr Surg 1994;94(2):388–93.

16. Marten TJ. High SMAS facelift: combined single flap lifting of the jawline, cheek, and midface. Clin Plast Surg 2008;35(4):569–603 vi-vii.

17. Feldman JJ. Neck lift. St Louis (MO): Quality Medical; 2006. p. 1–152.

18. Lambros V, Stuzin JM. The cross-cheek depression: surgical cause and effect in the development of the "joker line" and its treatment. Plast Reconstr Surg 2008;122(5):1543–52.

19. Hamra ST. Frequent face lift sequelae: hollow eyes and the lateral sweep: cause and repair. Plast Reconstr Surg 1998;102(5):1658–66.

20. Tonnard P, Verpaele A, Monstrey S, et al. Minimal access cranial suspension lift: a modified S-lift. Plast Reconstr Surg 2002;109(6):2074–86.

21. Hamra ST. The deep-plane rhytidectomy. Plast Reconstr Surg 1990;86(1):53–61 [discussion: 62–3].

22. Jacono AA, Parikh SS. The minimal access deep plane extended vertical facelift. Aesthet Surg J 2011;31(8):874–90.

23. Jacono AA, Ransom ER. Patient-specific rhytidectomy: finding the angle of maximal rejuvenation. Aesthet Surg J 2012;32(7):804–13.

24. Shah AR, Rosenberg D. Defining the facial extent of the platysma muscle: a review of 71 consecutive face-lifts. Arch Facial Plast Surg 2009;11(6):405–8.

25. Fogli A, Desouches C. Less invasive face-lifting: platysma anchoring techniques. Clin Plast Surg 2008;35(4):519–29, vi.

26. Siwani R, Friedman O. Anatomic evaluation of the vertical face-lift in cadavers. JAMA Facial Plast Surg 2013;15(6):422–7.

27. Alghoul M, Codner MA. Retaining ligaments of the face: review of anatomy and clinical applications. Aesthet Surg J 2013;33(6):769–82.

28. Furnas DW. The retaining ligaments of the cheek. Plast Reconstr Surg 1989;83(1):11–6.

29. Mendelson BC. Extended sub-SMAS dissection and cheek elevation. Clin Plast Surg 1995;22(2):325–39.

30. Stuzin JM, Baker TJ, Gordon HL. The relationship of the superficial and deep facial fascias: relevance to rhytidectomy and aging. Plast Reconstr Surg 1992;89(3):441–9 [discussion: 450–1].

31. Mendelson BC. Correction of the nasolabial fold: extended SMAS dissection with periosteal fixation. Plast Reconstr Surg 1992;89(5):822–33 [discussion: 834–5].

32. Muzaffar AR, Mendelson BC, Adams WP Jr. Surgical anatomy of the ligamentous attachments of the lower lid and lateral canthus. Plast Reconstr Surg 2002;110(3):873–84 [discussion: 897–911].

33. Ozdemir R, et al. Anatomicohistologic study of the retaining ligaments of the face and use in face lift: retaining ligament correction and SMAS plication. Plast Reconstr Surg 2002;110(4):1134–47 [discussion: 1148–9].

34. Gosain AK. Surgical anatomy of the facial nerve. Clin Plast Surg 1995;22(2):241–51.

35. Mendelson BC, Muzaffar AR, Adams WP Jr. Surgical anatomy of the midcheek and malar mounds. Plast Reconstr Surg 2002;110(3):885–96 [discussion: 897–911].

36. Moss CJ, Mendelson BC, Taylor GI. Surgical anatomy of the ligamentous attachments in the temple and periorbital regions. Plast Reconstr Surg 2000;105(4):1475–90 [discussion: 1491–8].

37. Owsley JQ, Agarwal CA. Safely navigating around the facial nerve in three dimensions. Clin Plast Surg 2008;35(4):469–77, v.

38. Stuzin JM, Wagstrom L, Kawamoto HK, et al. Anatomy of the frontal branch of the facial nerve: the significance of the temporal fat pad. Plast Reconstr Surg 1989;83(2):265–71.

39. Trussler AP, Stephan P, Hatef D, et al. The frontal branch of the facial nerve across the zygomatic arch: anatomical relevance of the high-SMAS technique. Plast Reconstr Surg 2010;125(4):1221–9.

40. Tzafetta K, Terzis JK. Essays on the facial nerve: part I. Microanatomy. Plast Reconstr Surg 2010;125(3):879–89.

41. Alghoul M, Bitik O, McBride J, et al. Relationship of the zygomatic facial nerve to the retaining ligaments of the face: the Sub-SMAS danger zone. Plast Reconstr Surg 2013;131(2):245e–52e.

42. Bosse J, Papillon J. Surgical anatomy of the SMAS at the malar region. In: Transactions of the IX International Congress of Plastic and Reconstructive Surgery. New York: McGraw-Hill; 1987. p. 348–9.

43. Mendelson BC. Anatomic study of the retaining ligaments of the face and applications for facial rejuvenation. Aesthetic Plast Surg 2013;37(3):513–5.

44. Rossell-Perry P, Paredes-Leandro P. Anatomic study of the retaining ligaments of the face and applications for facial rejuvenation. Aesthetic Plast Surg 2013;37(3):504–12.

45. Wong CH, Mendelson B. Facial soft-tissue spaces and retaining ligaments of the midcheek: defining the premaxillary space. Plast Reconstr Surg 2013;132(1):49–56.

46. McGregor M. Face lift techniques. Presented at the 1st Annual Meeting of the California Society of Plastic Surgeons. Yosemite, 1959.

47. Jacono AA, Parikh SS, Kennedy WA. Anatomical comparison of platysmal tightening using superficial musculoaponeurotic system plication vs deep-plane rhytidectomy techniques. Arch Facial Plast Surg 2011;13(6):395–7.

48. Mustoe TA, Rawlani V, Zimmerman H. Modified deep plane rhytidectomy with a lateral approach to the neck: an alternative to submental incision and dissection. Plast Reconstr Surg 2011;127(1):357–70.

49. Jacono AA, Rousso JJ. The modern minimally invasive face lift: has it replaced the traditional access

approach? Facial Plast Surg Clin North Am 2013; 21(2):171–89.

50. Brandt MG, Hassa A, Roth K, et al. Biomechanical properties of the facial retaining ligaments. Arch Facial Plast Surg 2012;14(4):289–94.

51. Langevin CJ, Engel S, Zins JE. Mandibular ligament revisited. Paper presented at: Ohio Valley Society of Plastic Surgery Annual Meeting. Cleveland, May 17, 2008.

52. Baker DC. Minimal incision rhytidectomy (short scar face lift) with lateral SMASectomy: evolution and application. Aesthet Surg J 2001;21(1):14–26.

53. Rees TD, Woodsmith D. Cosmetic facial surgery. Philadelphia: Saunders; 1973. p. 203.

54. Fuente del Campo A. Midline platysma muscular overlap for neck restoration. Plast Reconstr Surg 1998;102(5):1710–4 [discussion: 1715].

55. Guyuron B, Sadek EY, Ahmadian R. A 26-year experience with vest-over-pants technique platysmarrhaphy. Plast Reconstr Surg 2010;126(3):1027–34.

56. Feldman JJ. Corset platysmaplasty. Plast Reconstr Surg 1990;85(3):333–43.

57. Lee MK, Sepahdari A, Cohen M. Radiologic measurement of submandibular gland ptosis. Facial Plast Surg 2013;29(4):316–20.

58. DC B. Face lift with submandibular gland and digastric muscle resection: radical neck rhytidectomy. Aesthet Surg J 2006;26:85–92.

59. Cardoso de Castro C. The changing role of platysma in face lifting. Plast Reconstr Surg 2000; 105(2):764–75 [discussion: 776–7].

60. Byrd HS, Burt JD. Dimensional approach to rhinoplasty: perfecting the esthetic balance between the nose and chin. In: Gunter J, Rohrich RJ, Adams WP, editors. Dallas rhinoplasty: nasal surgery by the masters. St Louis (MO): Quality Medical Publishing; 2002. p. 117–31.

61. Courtiss EH. Suction lipectomy of the neck. Plast Reconstr Surg 1985;76(6):882–9

62. Rohrich RJ, Rios JL, Smith PD, et al. Neck rejuvenation revisited. Plast Reconstr Surg 2006;118(5):1251–63.

63. Marten TJ. Facelift. Planning and technique. Clin Plast Surg 1997;24(2):269–308.

64. Aston SJ. The FAME technique. Paper presented at: Symposium on the Aging Face, Laguna Niguel, Jan 14–15, 1993.

65. Aston SJ. Facelift with SMAS technique and FAME. In: Aston SJ, Steinbrech DS, Walden JL, editors. Aesthetic plast surg, 1. London: Saunders Elsevier; 2009. p. 73–85.

66. Adamson PA, Cormier R, Tropper GJ, et al. Cervicofacial liposuction: results and controversies. J Otolaryngol 1990;19(4):267–73.

67. Bank DE, Perez MI. Skin retraction after liposuction in patients over the age of 40. Dermatol Surg 1999; 25(9):673–6.

68. Chrisman BB. Liposuction with facelift surgery. Dermatol Clin 1990;8(3):501–22.

69. Daher JC, Cosac OM, Domingues S. Face-lift: the importance of redefining facial contours through facial liposuction. Ann Plast Surg 1988;21(1):1–10.

70. Dedo DD. Liposuction of the head and neck. Otolaryngol Head Neck Surg 1987;97(6):591–2.

71. Goodstein WA. Superficial liposculpture of the face and neck. Plast Reconstr Surg 1996;98(6):988–96 [discussion: 997–8].

72. Grotting JC, Beckenstein MS. Cervicofacial rejuvenation using ultrasound-assisted lipectomy. Plast Reconstr Surg 2001;107(3):847–55.

73. Jacob CI, Berkes BJ, Kaminer MS. Liposuction and surgical recontouring of the neck: a retrospective analysis. Dermatol Surg 2000;26(7):625–32.

74. Koehler J. Complications of neck liposuction and submentoplasty. Oral Maxillofac Surg Clin North Am 2009;21(1):43–52, vi.

75. O'Ryan F, Schendel S, Poor D. Submental-submandibular suction lipectomy: indications and surgical technique. Oral Surg Oral Med Oral Pathol 1989; 67(2):117–25.

76. de Castro CC. The anatomy of the platysma muscle. Plast Reconstr Surg 1980;66(5):680–3.

77. McKinney P. Management of platysmal bands. Plast Reconstr Surg 2002;110(3):982–4.

78. Perkins SW, Gibson FB. Use of submentoplasty to enhance cervical recontouring in face-lift surgery. Arch Otolaryngol Head Neck Surg 1993;119(2):179–83.

79. Aston SJ. Platysma-SMAS cervicofacial rhytidoplasty. Clin Plast Surg 1983;10(3):507–20.

80. Adamson PA, Moran ML. Historical trends in surgery for the aging face. Facial Plast Surg 1993; 9(2):133–42.

81. Baker DC. Complications of cervicofacial rhytidectomy. Clin Plast Surg 1983;10(3):543–62.

82. Baker DC. Deep dissection rhytidectomy: a plea for caution. Plast Reconstr Surg 1994;93(7):1498–9.

83. Rees TD, Aston SJ. A clinical evaluation of the results of submusculo-aponeurotic dissection and fixation in face lifts. Plast Reconstr Surg 1977; 60(6):851–9.

84. WH B. Extended posterior rhytidectomy. Facial Plast Surg Clin North Am 1993;1:215.

85. Baker TJ, Gordon HL, Mosienko P. Rhytidectomy: a statistical analysis. Plast Reconstr Surg 1977;59(1):24–30.

86. Chang S, Pusic A, Rohrich RJ. A systematic review of comparison of efficacy and complication rates among face-lift techniques. Plast Reconstr Surg 2011;127(1):423–33.

87. Matarasso A, Elkwood A, Rankin M, et al. National plastic surgery survey: face lift techniques and complications. Plast Reconstr Surg 2000;106(5):1185–95 [discussion: 1196].

88. McKinney P, Katrana DJ. Prevention of injury to the great auricular nerve during rhytidectomy. Plast Reconstr Surg 1980;66(5):675–9.

89. Rohrich RJ, Taylor NS, Ahmad J, et al. Great auricular nerve injury, the "subauricular band" phenomenon, and the periauricular adipose compartments. Plast Reconstr Surg 2011;127(2):835–43.

90. Stuzin JM. MOC-PSSM CME article: face lifting. Plast Reconstr Surg 2008;121(Suppl 1):1–19.

91. Rees TD, Aston SJ. Complications of rhytidectomy. Clin Plast Surg 1978;5(1):109–19.

92. Owsley JQ Jr. SMAS-platysma face lift. Plast Reconstr Surg 1983;71(4):573–6.

93. Lemmon ML, Hamra ST. Skoog rhytidectomy: a five-year experience with 577 patients. Plast Reconstr Surg 1980;65(3):283–97.

94. Prado A, Andrades P, Danilla S, et al. A clinical retrospective study comparing two short-scar face lifts: minimal access cranial suspension versus lateral SMASectomy. Plast Reconstr Surg 2006;117(5): 1413–25 [discussion: 1426–7].

95. Adamson PA, Dahiya R, Litner J. Midface effects of the deep-plane vs the superficial musculoaponeurotic system plication face-lift. Arch Facial Plast Surg 2007;9(1):9–11.

96. Kamer FM, Frankel AS. SMAS rhytidectomy versus deep plane rhytidectomy: an objective comparison. Plast Reconstr Surg 1998;102(3): 878–81.

97. Barton FE Jr. Aesthetic surgery of the face and neck. Aesthet Surg J 2009;29(6):449–63 [quiz: 464–6].

Complications/Sequelae of Neck Rejuvenation

Rami K. Batniji, MD

KEYWORDS

- Neck lift • Cervicofacial rhytidectomy • Complications

KEY POINTS

- Expanding hematoma may result in skin flap necrosis and/or airway compromise; therefore, immediate evacuation followed by control of hemostasis is recommended.
- Hematoma or seroma may result in induration; induration may resolve spontaneously, may require conservative treatment with injection of steroid and massage, or may result in skin contour irregularities that may benefit from revision surgery.
- The most commonly injured nerve is the great auricular nerve, and the most commonly injured motor nerve is the marginal mandibular branch of the facial nerve.
- Although infection following neck lift surgery is rare, the rate of methicillin-resistant *Staphylococcus aureus* infection is on the rise and should be considered in the differential diagnosis of infection following neck lift surgery.
- Persistent platysmal bands are treated with either botulinum toxin, submentoplasty, or corset platysmaplasty.

INTRODUCTION

Neck lift surgery performed in isolation or in conjunction with a facelift provides a more youthful cervicomental angle. Complications related to neck lift surgery vary from contour irregularities that may improve with time or conservative measures, to contour irregularities that persist and may benefit from delayed surgical intervention, to expanding hematomas that require immediate surgical intervention. This article reviews complications of neck lift surgery and their etiologies, methods to minimize the incidence of these complications, and management.

HEMATOMA

The rate of hematoma in neck lift is approximately 3% and does not increase with use of a deep plane procedure.[1] Risk factors include hypertension, male gender, use of certain medications/ supplements/herbal/homeopathic medications, including aspirin, nonsteroidal anti-inflammatory medications, fish oil, gingko biloba, and melatonin, to name a few.[2] In an effort to minimize this risk, proper perioperative management of hypertension is essential, as well as avoidance of medications/ supplements/homeopathic medications that may increase bleeding. In patients with a history of easy bruising, preoperative evaluation of coagulation studies may reveal an underlying coagulopathy, thalassemia should be suspected as a potential issue in patients of Mediterranean descent and history of easy bruising. A meta-analysis demonstrated no statistically significant benefit from the use of tissue sealants in face-lift surgery; however, tissue sealants may be useful for patients at high risk for hematoma formation.[3] A prospective randomized controlled trial demonstrated no influence on postoperative hematoma by the use of drains in cervicofacial rhytidectomy; however, this study did show a significant reduction in bruising with the use

Disclosures: None.
Batniji Facial Plastic Surgery, 361 Hospital Road, Suite 329, Newport Beach, CA 92663, USA
E-mail address: ramikbatniji@gmail.com

Facial Plast Surg Clin N Am 22 (2014) 317–320
http://dx.doi.org/10.1016/j.fsc.2014.01.007
1064-7406/14/$ – see front matter © 2014 Elsevier Inc. All rights reserved.

of drains, which may be useful in patients at high risk for hematoma following surgery.[4] A retrospective study found the use of drains during the first 24 hours after cervicofacial rhytidectomy significantly decreases the rate of seroma formation, and, to a lesser extent, hematoma formation.[5] If an expanding hematoma is encountered in the postoperative period, immediate evacuation of the hematoma and exploration of the operative site for hemostasis control are essential due to the potential for airway compromise and skin flap necrosis. If a small, nonexpanding hematoma develops in the postoperative period, needle aspiration and compression dressing, followed by close observation and further needle aspiration as needed may be sufficient; a postoperative seroma may be managed similarly. If the hematoma is organized, and, as such, not amenable to needle aspiration, then one may consider partial opening of incision site, suctioning of organized hematoma, closure of incision site, and placement of a compression dressing.

INDURATION

A seroma or small hematoma may result in induration. If induration occurs, it may be treated with massage and/or injection of triamcinolone 10 mg/mL approximately 4 weeks after surgery. Triamcinolone injection may cause subdermal atrophy and/or skin hyperpigmentation; placement of the injection deep into the subcutaneous plane and diluting the steroid may minimize these risks. Usually, these conservative measures and the passage of time allow for resolution of the induration and address the induration without producing a long-term skin contour irregularity. If a skin contour irregularity persists 6 to 12 months after the original surgery, it is reasonable to consider a surgery that would involve a wide undermining of skin to provide a second chance for improved skin contraction.

SKIN CONTOUR IRREGULARITIES

Skin contour irregularities after neck lift surgery have several possible etiologies. Overzealous liposuction of fat superficial to the platysma muscle may result in skin contour irregularities. If the contour irregularity is only a concavity, then 1 possible solution is injection of filler, such as hyaluronic acid, or fat grafting into the concavity. Occasionally, this overzealous liposuctioning may lead to adherence of denuded dermis directly onto the platysma muscle, leading to contour irregularities. In such instances, undermining of skin off of the platysma muscle and redraping offer some

improvement, and fat grafting may provide additional improvement. During liposuction of fat superficial to the platysma muscle, consider using small cannulas, turning the hole of the cannula away from the dermis, and performing judicious rather than excessive liposuction.

Skin contour irregularities at the postauricular region may be related to insufficient undermining of skin, which may be seen in short scar procedures. Rohrich and colleagues[6] named this irregularity a "subauricular band" and described it as a lateral neck band with skin contour irregularities along the posterior aspect of the sternocleidomastoid muscle. Proper undermining of skin will help prevent this complication. If this complication occurs, then release of this band with complete undermining of the involved and surrounding areas will minimize the irregularity.

NERVE INJURY

The great auricular nerve is the most commonly injured nerve during cervicofacial rhytidectomy. Meticulous, precise dissection in the region inferior to McKinney point, where the great auricular nerve is more superficial and, as such, more susceptible to potential injury, will minimize this risk. In addition to ear numbness, transection of the great auricular nerve may lead to formation of a neuroma; if a neuroma develops and presents as a painful superficial mass, then surgical excision of the neuroma is warranted.[7] The marginal mandibular branch of the facial nerve is the most commonly injured motor nerve and results in weakness of the ipsilateral hemi-lower lip due to denervation of the depressor anguli oris, depressor labii inferioris, and mentalis muscles. In most cases, it is a traction injury that is not permanent, and function eventually returns to normal within weeks or a few months. Injury to the cervical branch of the facial nerve may result in the clinical presentation of pseudoparalysis of the marginal mandibular nerve; the cervical branch of the facial nerve injury can be distinguished from marginal mandibular nerve injury by the fact that the patient will be able to evert the lower lip because of a functioning mentalis muscle.[8]

INFECTION

Infection following cervicofacial rhytidectomy is not common, with a reported incidence of 0.6%; however, methicillin-resistant S aureus (MRSA) infections are on the rise.[9] It behooves the facial plastic surgeon to review the patient's past medical and surgical histories to identify potential risk factors for either community-acquired or health care-associated MRSA. Patients at risk include those with a history of previous hospitalization, diabetes, smoking, obesity, and employment as a health care worker, and/or recent antimicrobial therapy. As MRSA is on the rise, screening protocols including preoperative cultures of the nose, throat, groin, and any existing wounds have increasingly become implemented at surgery centers and hospitals. In those cases with MRSA colonization and no clinical signs of infection, patients are treated with mupirocin nasal ointment 3 times daily, 2% triclosan washes twice daily for 5 days and chlorhexidine mouthwash 2 to 3 times daily for 5 days.[10] Some practices have eliminated screening and started treating all patients with the mupirocin nasal swabs preoperatively. Other preoperative and intraoperative measures to minimize risk of infection include preparing with chlorhexidine gluconate, administering prophylactic antibiotics within 1 hour of surgery, providing supplemental oxygen, and maintaining normothermia and normoglycemia. If a purulent infection is identified after surgery, consider incision and drainage, obtaining cultures, and placing the patient on broad-spectrum antibiotics until availability of culture results. Timely identification of infection and incision and drainage is emphasized in a case report of death caused by septic dual sinus thrombosis attributable to community-acquired MRSA.[11]

PERSISTENT PLATYSMAL BANDS

Persistent platysmal bands may result from inadequate correction or failure of plication sutures. A nonsurgical treatment of persistent platysmal bands is injection of botulinum toxin.[12] Perkins and Gibson[13] described the use of submentoplasty as a secondary procedure to address persistent platysmal bands, submental fullness, and excess submental skin. Through a submental incision, wide local undermining of skin is performed. A Kelly clamp is used to grasp the platysma and excess tissue contributing to submental fullness; the tissue and muscle clamped by the instrument are then resected, and the medial edges of platysma muscle are plicated with interrupted, buried suture. Another option is a corset platysmaplasty via a submental incision as described by Feldman.[14]

EARLOBE DISTORTION/PIXIE EAR DEFORMITY

During neck lift surgery, if too much tension is placed at the earlobe attachment to the skin flap, migration of the earlobe attachment point from a posterior cephalad position to an anterior caudal position may occur, resulting in a pixie ear deformity. A method to minimize the formation of this deformity is tension-free closure of skin at the time of initial surgery. One method of correcting a pixie ear deformity involves releasing the tethered lobule by cutting the subcutaneous scar holding the earlobe down and advancing the infralobular and postauricular skin flap in an upward direction through an incision that involves the lobule and extends into the postauricular sulcus.[15]

PTOTIC AND/OR LARGE SUBMANDIBULAR GLAND

Fullness in the submandibular triangle of the neck following neck lift surgery may be related to a normal-sized, ptotic submandibular gland or a large gland that may or may not be ptotic. Although the ptotic submandibular gland may be hidden behind a heavy neck with significant adipose tissue, palpation of the neck during consultation may provide the surgeon with information regarding the position and size of the submandibular gland. Various techniques have been described to address the ptotic submandibular gland. At the time of neck lift surgery, a submandibular sling suture from midline-to-mastoid may assist in repositioning the ptotic submandibular gland; however, patients may complain of tightness in the neck due to these sutures.[16] In patients with normal-sized, ptotic submandibular glands, Guyuron and colleagues[17] reported effective long-term results in the treatment of submandibular gland fullness with a suture passed through the deep temporal fascia, the gland, and the medial surface of the mandible in a basket fashion. Some advocate partial resection of the gland.[18] Potential risks associated with any resection of the submandibular gland include bleeding, injury to nerves (marginal mandibular branch of facial nerve, hypoglaossal nerve, lingual nerve, and mylohyoid nerve), xerostomia, sialoma, and hollowness in the submandibular triangle secondary to over-resection of the gland. If a patient who underwent a neck lift has a fullness in the neck due to the gland and is interested in less invasive procedures to address this fullness, one may consider the use of botulinum toxin into the gland to shrink the gland or injection of filler to camouflage the bulge caused by the gland.[19]

HAIRLINE DISTORTION

In neck lift surgery, the postauricular incision may be carried within the postauricular sulcus or on the posterior surface of the concha near the postauricular sulcus. From there, the incision may be extended into the occipital hairline or along the occipital hairline. In an effort to minimize hairline distortion, it is imperative to match up the hairline if the incision is carried into the hairline. If the incision is carried along the hairline, one may consider beveling the incision to allow the growth of hair follicles through the incision site or a w-plasty to minimize the appearance of a scar. Essential to minimal appearance of scar is tension-free closure of skin.[20] If the occipital hairline is displaced posteriorly, one option is a hair restoration procedure to restore a more natural occipital hairline.

SUMMARY

Rejuvenation of the neck with neck lift surgery can provide a more youthful cervicomental angle. Thorough preoperative assessment of the patient's anatomy, medications, and medical history, as well as meticulous surgical technique and postoperative care, may assist in minimizing complications in neck lift surgery. If a complication occurs, timely and appropriate management of that complication with empathy and compassion is recommended.

REFERENCES

1. Nahai F, Bryce A. Deep plane procedures in the neck. In: Aston SJ, Steinbrech D, Walden J, editors. Aesthetic plastic surgery. New York: Elsevier; 2009. p. 231–42.
2. Wong WW, Gabriel A, Maxwell GP, et al. Bleeding risks of herbal, homeopathic, and dietary supplements: a hidden nightmare for plastic surgeons? Aesthet Surg J 2012;32(3):332–46.
3. Por YC, Shi L, Samuel M, et al. Use of tissue sealants in face-lifts: a meta-analysis. Aesthetic Plast Surg 2009;33(3):336–9.
4. Jones BM, Grover R, Hamilton S. The efficacy of surgical drainage in cervicofacial rhytidectomy: a prospective, randomized, controlled trial. Plast Reconstr Surg 2007;120(1):263–70.
5. Perkins SW, Williams JD, Macdonald K, et al. Prevention of seromas and hematomas after face-lift surgery with the use of postoperative vacuum drains. Arch Otolaryngol Head Neck Surg 1997; 123(7):743–5.
6. Rohrich RJ, Taylor NS, Ahmad J, et al. Great auricular nerve injury, the "subauricular band" phenomenon,
and the periauricular adipose compartments. Plast Reconstr Surg 2011;127(2):835–43.
7. De Chalian T, Nahai F. Amputation neuromas of the great auricular nerve after rhytidectomy. Ann Plast Surg 1995;35(3):297–9.
8. Daane SP, Owsley JQ. Incidence of cervical branch injury with "marginal mandibular nerve pseudo-paralysis" in patients undergoing face lift. Plast Reconstr Surg 2003;111(7):2414–8.
9. Zoumalan RA, Rosenberg DB. Methicillin-resistant *Staphylcoccus aureus*-positive surgical site infections in face-lift surgery. Arch Facial Plast Surg 2008;10(2):116–23.
10. Malde DJ, Abidia A, McCollum C, et al. The success of routine MRSA screening in vascular surgery: a nine year review. Int Angiol 2006;25(2):204–8.
11. Sifri CD, Solenski NJ. Fatal septic thrombosis of the superior sagittal sinus after face-lift surgery caused by community-associated methicillin-resistant *Staphylococcus aureus*. Plast Reconstr Surg 2009;11(2):142–5.
12. Kane MA. Nonsurgical treatment of platysma bands with injection of botulinum toxin a revisited. Plast Reconstr Surg 2003;112(Suppl 5):125S–6S.
13. Perkins SW, Gibson FB. Use of submentoplasty to enhance cervical recontouring in face-lift surgery. Arch Otolaryngol Head Neck Surg 1993;119(2): 179–83.
14. Feldman JJ. Correcting problems from a previous neck lift. In: Feldman JJ, editor. Neck lift. St Louis (MO): Quality Medical Publishing, Inc; 2006. p. 497–519.
15. Feldman JJ. Earlobe shaping. In: Feldman JJ, editor. Neck lift. St Louis (MO): Quality Medical Publishing, Inc; 2006. p. 473–95.
16. Nahai F. Reconsidering neck suspension sutures. Aesthet Surg J 2004;24(4):365–7.
17. Guyuron B, Jackowe D, Iamphongsai S. Basket submandibular gland suspension. Plast Reconstr Surg 2008;122(3):938–43.
18. Feldman JJ. Submandibular salivary gland bulges. In: Feldman JJ, editor. Neck lift. St Louis (MO): Quality Medical Publishing, Inc; 2006. p. 397–448.
19. Connell BF. Male facelift. Aesthet Surg J 2002;22(4): 385–96.
20. Kridel RW, Liu ES. Techniques for creating inconspicuous face-lift scars: avoiding visible incisions and loss of temporal hair. Arch Facial Plast Surg 2003;5(4):325–33.

Index

Note: Page numbers of article titles are in **boldface** type.

A

Ablation threshold, of biologic tissue, 209

Ablative CO_2 laser, in neck skin rejuvenation, 205–206, 208, 210–214
    fractional vs., 207. See also *Fractional CO_2 laser.*
    pulse duration effect on treatment density, 210–212

Absorption spectra, for Nd:YAG fiber lasers, 218

Adipocytes, Nd:YAG fiber laser interactions with, 218–219

Adiposity. See *Fat/fatty tissue.*

Adjunctive procedures, in neck rejuvenation, **231–242**
    chin augmentation as, 234, 236–240
        expanded polytetrafluorethylene in, 234
        grafts for, 234
        indications for, 234
        intraoral approach to implant placement, 237
        mersilene mesh in, 237
        outcomes of, 238–240
        polyamide mesh in, 234, 236
        porous polyethylene in, 234
        post procedure care of, 238
        silicone rubber in, 237
        submental approach to implant placement, 238
    fibrin sealants as, 231–236
        authors' experience with, 232–233
        coagulation cascade and, 231–232
        drains vs., 231
        historical use of, 232
        outcomes of, 234–236
        procedure for, 233–234
    for platysma, 248–250
        laser skin resurfacing as, 248–249
        neuromodulators as, 248
        submental liposuction as, 249–250
    hyoid bone position and, 239–240
    introduction to, 231
    key points of, 231
    Nd:YAG interstitial fiber laser as, 217–218, 224, 226–228
    submandibular gland ptosis and, 238–239
    summary overview of, 240–241
    in vertical neck lifting, 292
        submental, 303–304, 309, 311, 313

Advance-and-spread technique, in extended SMAS rhytidectomy, 260–261

Aesthetics, of neck lift, 285–286
    with intense focused ultrasound, 200
    of neck rejuvenation, 171, 174, 180, 253
    with deep-plane approach, 274, 280–281

Aging neck, anatomy and physiology of, **161–170**
    aging patterns and, 161–162
    by structure, 161–169
        deep plane, 169, 270–271
    cartilaginous structures in, 169
    cervical fascia in, 163–164
        superficial vs. deep, 163–164
    cervicomental angle in, 161, 163, 166–167, 169, 269
    hyoid in, 169
    introduction to, 161
    key points of, 161
    lymphatics in, 165
    mandible in, 169
    platysma in, 165–166
    radiographic imaging indications for, 169, 244, 257
    skin in, 162–164
        histologic features of, 163
    subcutaneous fat in, 164–165
    subplatysmal deep compartment in, 166–169
        deep plane defined by, 166–167, 271
        digastric muscle and, 167
        facial nerve and, 168–169
        great auricular nerve and, 168
        sternocleidomastoid muscle and, 161–162, 164, 168
        submandibular glands and, 168
        subplatysmal fat and, 166–167
    summary overview of, 169–170
    superficial muscular aponeurotic system in, 165, 270–271
    triangular sections in, 162
    youthful neck vs., 161–162, 164, 171, 174, 243, 269–270, 285
    classification of. See *Aging patterns.*
    lines in, 172. See also *Banding.*
    rejuvenation of. See *Neck skin rejuvenation; Rhytidectomy.*
    preoperative evaluation of, **171–176**
        clinical neck procedure evaluation and, 173–175
        history taking in, 172–173, 181
        physical examination in, 173–175
        introduction to, 171–173

http://dx.doi.org/10.1016/S1064-7406(14)00026-1
1064-7406/14/$ – see front matter © 2014 Elsevier Inc. All rights reserved.

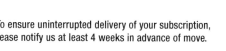